THE SAVE-

Proven Protection From Six Of The Most Serious Diseases Of

Civilization™

THE

SAVE-YOUR-LIFE

DIET

Proven protection from six of the most serious diseases of civilization™

DAVID REUBEN, M.D.

The Save-Your-Life Diet
Revised Edition
Copyright © 2014 Tulipanes Cristalinos del Oeste, S.A.
All rights reserved.
Cover design by: **dbyD**™

Other Books By David Reuben, M.D.

Everything You Always Wanted To Know About Sex But Were Afraid To Ask™

Any Woman Can! *Love and sexual fulfillment for the single, widowed, divorced, and married*™

How To Get More Out of Sex *Than you ever thought you could*™

The Save-Your-Life Diet *Proven protection from six of the most serious diseases of civilization*™

The Save-Your-Life Diet High Fiber Cookbook™

Everything You Always Wanted To Know About Nutrition™

Dr. David Reuben's Mental First-Aid Manual *Instant Relief! ... from 23 of life's worst problems*™

The Quick Weight-Gain Program *Safe, easy weight-gain for every age and situation*™

Everything You Always Wanted To Know About Sex But Were Afraid To Ask™ ALL NEW EDITION

Psychiatric Hospital *Where insanity meets reality ... and reality is insane*™

The Diet of Diets *The Diet that never disappoints!*™

The Chinese Secret *How to save yourself from breast and prostate cancer ... and enjoy sex like never before!*™

Table of Contents

An Open Letter to My Fellow Physicians

David Reuben, M.D.
author@davidreubenmd.com

Dear Colleague:

A lot of things have happened since this book topped the best seller lists in 1975. In those days it was a long hard struggle to convince anyone, including some of my colleagues, that a high fiber, low fat diet, was effective in preventing and/or treating the following eleven diseases:

> Heart attacks (myocardial infarcts)
> Reducing the risk of colon cancer
> Blood clots in the legs spreading to the lungs (phlebitis
> to pulmonary embolism)
> Appendicitis
> Constipation
> Diverticular disease
> Irritable bowel syndrome
> Hemorrhoids
> Varicose veins
> High levels of serum cholesterol
> Obesity
> High blood pressure

And of course, now there is no doubt that a high fiber diet can help prevent all those conditions and others as well. Therefore, the role of this book in preventive medicine is far more important than ever before. Your patients are deluged with a flood of information every day emanating from the Internet. A lot of it is amateur and incorrect. This book can provide a source of easy-to-read and absolutely factual information for your patients which will save you time by reinforcing your diagnosis and treatment and increasing patient compliance.

If you have any questions or comments I would be delighted to hear from you. And you can be sure I will reply promptly and personally.

With very best wishes for your continued success,

Fraternally yours,

David Reuben, M.D.

Why I Wrote This Book

For five years I watched my father die slowly of cancer of the colon. I made sure he had the finest doctors in the country and the most advanced treatment available. It didn't make any difference.

The slow-growing cancer relentlessly destroyed him. No one could tell me the cause of his malignancy, no one could tell me how it could have been prevented, and the best treatment modern medicine could offer was essentially the same as that used in 1900. The surgeons cut out the tumor and most of his large intestine; they relocated his anus to his lower abdomen, which caused him great emotional trauma. In spite of devoted doctors and massive medical costs, he died.

Shortly after his death, I noticed a small article in one of the medical journals suggesting that restoring roughage to the modern diet might be beneficial in treating constipation, hemorrhoids, and "irritable colon"—three conditions that are annoying but hardly life-threatening. But I also knew that these three conditions have a statistical correlation with cancer of the colon. So I followed up the article, and for the next four years I read nearly every bit of scientific material written on the role of roughage in human disease. I am now convinced that not only could my father's life have been saved, but millions of other cancer victims would be alive today if they had simply been able to add a few cents worth of fiber to their daily diet.

I must admit that when I first began my research I had the usual physician's skepticism. The articles—even in the medical journals—

seemed reminiscent of those advocating wheat germ, blackstrap molasses, and yogurt.

But now that over five thousand unassailable articles have been published in respected medical journals around the world confirming and reconfirming the validity of the findings, there seems little doubt that adding the missing roughage to our daily diet provides real protection from:

Heart Attacks (Myocardial Infarcts)
Reducing the risk of colon cancer
Blood clots in the legs spreading to the lungs (phlebitis
to pulmonary embolism)
Appendicitis
Constipation
Diverticular disease
Irritable bowel syndrome
Hemorrhoids
Varicose veins
High levels of serum cholesterol
Obesity
High blood pressure

I know that this sounds like the claims on a bottle of Vegetable Tonic—and that worried me until I saw each element of protection validated and revalidated in the most rigorously scientific studies.

This is the most exciting medical story of this century — and I feel that by telling it simply, directly, and honestly I can benefit a lot of people except of course ... my father.

Important Message

This book does not constitute medical treatment or medical advice. Do not undertake any medical program unless until you have had a thorough examination and consultation with your physician. As with any diet program, if at any time during the program you experience any discomfort or serious symptoms consult your physician immediately.

1

How To Prevent Heart Attacks And The Major Forms Of Cancer

Consider a medical Garden of Eden. Imagine a society where heart attacks don't exist, where a terrible form of death-dealing cancer is virtually unknown, where phlebitis and the resulting fatal blood clots in the lungs are almost unheard of. Think of a world where many of the petty ailments of modern society have been virtually eliminated—appendicitis, hemorrhoids, obesity, diverticulosis of the colon, and varicose veins. Is this the United States in the year 3000?

No. It's rural Africa today. It's a society and a way of life that has *almost completely avoided the major scourges of the modern world.* Most important of all, buried in the tribal life of these Africans is a secret that can make a better life for nearly every man and woman in America.

We all know—from the yearly newspaper stories— that life expectancy in the United States has increased dramatically in the past fifty years. **But few of us know how deceptive these statistics are.** The life expectancy number is bigger *but **not** because our general health is improving*—it's merely because fewer children now die before the age of five. (Life-expectancy calculations use a complex formula based on age at death of those who die each year to arrive at an expectancy figure for those still living. As more children survive longer —due to antibiotics, immunization, and better sanitation —the overall figure of "life expectancy" is *deceptively* increased.)

Actually, in some years even the official figure has been declining. That's because as each year passes, more Americans succumb to the two great destroyers, cancer and heart attacks. In addition, obesity, diverticular disease, and high blood pressure are also increasing. Worst of all, modern medicine seems to be helpless in stemming the tide.

The basic treatment of cancer has not changed since 1900: wait until the wildly multiplying cells take over part of the body and then desperately try to destroy the tissues or the organ they have invaded. The survival rates from cancer mirror our impotence.

And our progress in avoiding heart attacks isn't that impressive. In spite of spending trillions (that's right, *trillions*) on research and shiny electronic equipment, we are still helpless to prevent heart attacks in any meaningful way. We don't even know how to effectively *treat* a heart-attack victim—even the stent and by-pass surgery have not lived up to expectations.

The same applies to the other killers—high blood pressure, diverticulitis, obesity, and blood clots in the deep veins of the legs and lungs. Cause: unknown. Treatment: directed at symptoms, not at the basic cause. (The treatment for high blood pressure lowers the pressure, treatment for blood clots tries to dissolve the clots, treatment for obesity tries to suppress the appetite. But none of those treat the *underlying causes* of the conditions.)

In a tale that has all the excitement and suspense of a mystery story, a small group of British scientists made a series of discoveries that promises to remove— once and for all—these crippling and deadly diseases as threats to the health of our nation—and the entire world. The tracking of clues extends all the way from analyzing the lunch menu in an African village to studying bakery recipes in an English mill town in 1850.

Prosaically, it all began with an observation about the bowel movements of African villagers. English doctors working among the natives noticed that the Africans passed about one pound of fecal material per day. This was a startling contrast to the normal English bowel movement of less than four ounces!

There were other differences: the Africans' feces were bulky, soft, and almost completely odor-free; the British bowel movements were hard and compressed, and had a rotten, putrefied odor. To the average person a bowel movement is a source of embarrassment, the butt of infantile jokes, and the object of almost compulsive cleanliness. But to a physician the feces are an important source of information about one of the most essential functions of the human body—digestion.

Everything that happens to your body—or is going to happen to it—is dependent on the process of converting what you consume into the cells, tissues, and organs of your body. The process of digestion is complicated and still poorly understood in comparison to some other less important bodily processes. However, there are some highlights that are especially significant.

The processing of the food you eat, from the mouth through the stomach and intestines, is very similar to a mining process. If you consider your daily diet to be the raw ore, the goal of digestion is to extract the fat, protein, carbohydrates, vitamins, and minerals that your organism needs. Once that is accomplished, the sludge or tailings from the refining process must be disposed of. Scientists always considered this to be the least important part of the digestive process. In the colon or large intestine, water is absorbed, bacteria act on the residue (as a matter of fact, up to 30 percent of feces are composed of bacteria), and the powerful muscles of the colon compress the mass like a gigantic trash compacter. The resulting fecal contents are then expelled.

The medical investigators knew all that, but they were at a loss to explain why the Africans should produce four times as much fecal mass, odor-free and consistently soft and bulky. Their next discovery was even more puzzling—the food consumed by the Africans went from the dinner table to the bowel movement in as little as twenty-four hours! The average Englishman retained what he ate for a full three days, and some individual Britons took up to two weeks to fully process their food.

Intrigued by these findings, the researchers pressed on. They began to analyze the daily diets of the rural Africans and made even more fascinating discoveries—discoveries that open the door to freedom from incalculable suffering and expense for millions of people.

The average village dweller ate a diet that was pitiful by our standards. He consumed corn meal, beans, bananas, and potatoes. His daily food ration was notable in only one regard: it was extremely high in vegetable fiber. That's the part of plant material people eat but are unable to completely digest. It includes most of the things that stick in your teeth, make chewing hard and make vegetables difficult to consume: things like the bran on the grain of wheat, the strings in string beans, part of the oats in rolled oats, the skins of apples and potatoes, and all the rest. Because the Africans consumed so much of this fiber or "roughage," their food fairly raced through their digestive system. That much was interesting but certainly not exciting. When the Britishers summarized their findings, this was what they had:

Africans had more massive, heavier, less odoriferous bowel movements than Englishmen.

Africans moved their food through the body three times faster than Englishmen.

Africans ate about three times as much roughage or vegetable fiber as Englishmen.

That would have been material for an obscure article in a minor medical journal except—fortunately for the world—the British doctors didn't stop there. They began to look for other differences between the supposedly "deprived" Africans and their much more affluent English counterparts. What they found may be about to revolutionize modern medicine. Their discovery, I believe, is potentially more valuable than much of the multibillion dollar medical research conducted over the past half century. Their simple observations may save millions from the pain and suffering and death of heart attacks and cancer and avoid tens of billions of dollars' worth of surgery, hospital stays, and therapy.

After a painstaking analysis of countless medical records—comparing death and illness rates for various groups—this is what the researchers found:

1. Coronary heart disease, the cause of heart attacks which are *responsible for one-third of all deaths in the United States*, is virtually *unknown* in rural Africa.

2. Cancer of the colon and rectum, the second most common types of lethal cancer in the United States, is extremely rare in country-dwelling Africans.

3. Appendicitis, the most common abdominal surgical emergency in the United States, is almost never encountered among African villagers.

4. Hemorrhoids, that scourge of civilization, the cause of untold suffering and disability, is extremely rare among those eating the traditional African diet.

5. Among Americans, diverticulosis (pockets pouching out in the wall of the large intestine) is the most common disease of the colon; half of older Americans are its victims. Africans almost never get it.

6. Ten percent of all Americans have varicose veins. It is very unusual for a rural African to have this condition.

7. Phlebitis is an everyday cause of illness and suffering among Americans. Phlebitis (blood clots in the deep veins of the legs) is potentially lethal since at any moment the clots can shoot upward into the lungs and cause sudden death. Africans rarely are afflicted by this condition.

8. Obesity and overweight, those disabling and disfiguring conditions, affect 63% of Americans! Africans who adhere to their traditional diet *do not become overweight.*

These eight simple facts were almost too much for many sophisticated medical minds to absorb.

Could it be that the simple, almost inadequate diet of the Africans saved them from the half-dozen diseases that kill or cripple scores of millions in North America and Europe?

Could it be that our diet—packed with protein, enriched with vitamins and minerals, safeguarded by government standards—could be so deficient in some vital factor that it is filling our hospitals and cemeteries with victims of cancer and heart attacks?

Is it possible that almost a million American doctors, dedicated to removing cancerous organs, ministering to heart-attack victims, and operating on appendicitis, varicose veins, hemorrhoids, and diverticulosis could someday devote their attention to practicing the *preventive medicine* they all agree is more effective?

These questions had to be answered once and for all— not on the basis of wishful thinking, but by objective analysis of scientific facts. Maybe the observation that rural Africans were spared so much illness while the health of "modern" society was deteriorating could be explained on the basis of heredity.

Perhaps there was something in the genes of black Africans that provided them with immunity to these terrible diseases. The researchers continued their investigations. More tedious analysis of medical records around the world produced these findings:

1. Africans who adopt a *Western diet* gradually develop *Western diseases*. Obviously it takes some time for the conditions to become manifest, although appendicitis shows up first in Africans who drastically cut the amount of roughage in their diets. Gradually cancer of the colon, heart attacks, diverticulosis, and all the rest of the grim illnesses begin to follow.

2. Black Africans who come to the United States and adopt an American diet slowly succumb to these degenerative diseases. Within about thirty years the conditions begin to appear in alarming numbers.

Trying to explain the difference in susceptibility in terms of racial differences led up a blind alley in another respect. Native Japanese on a traditional diet are nearly as free from these conditions as African blacks. But when Japanese move to Hawaii and adopt a low-roughage diet there, they slowly begin to develop heart attacks and colon cancer in increasing amounts, along with the rest of the low-fiber diseases. Another bit of confirmatory evidence comes from the "Westernized" Japanese who still live in Japan but have adopted an American-style low-fiber diet. Their illness and death rate inevitably follows the American pattern.

Even Caucasians like Turks and Romanians relentlessly begin to succumb to the fiber deficiency diseases shortly after they relinquish their high-roughage traditional diets and eat the way Americans and Britons do.

Spurred on by these vital discoveries, the medical researchers began to analyze the modern American and British diets. What they found was an amazing chronicle of how so-called progress extracts its price. At the same time they discovered the means of potentially sparing all of us the disease and disability that has become an almost inevitable consequence of our way of life.

2

The One Deficiency In Our Modern Diet
That Is Killing Us

A s the original findings of those on-the-scene medical researchers were published in international medical journals, other scientists around the world turned their attention to the relationship between the epidemic of degenerative diseases and the diet of modern western-society men and women.

What they discovered was a shocking indictment of current nutritional practices. In effect, modern diets are glaringly deficient in that single substance that is related to a long and disease-free life. To put it bluntly, affluent Americans (and other Westerners) are eating a high-priced, high-prestige diet that leads them directly to cancer of the colon, heart attacks, obesity, and high blood pressure. In addition, the greater part of what was considered the "burdens of civilization"—hemorrhoids, varicose veins, diverticulosis, "irritable colon," appendicitis, and others—are *simply the result of a deficient diet*.

At this point there are two obstacles to understanding the problem.

First, how can a diet that is as rich and as varied as the typical American diet possibly be deficient?

The answer is this: our diet is neither as "rich" nor as "varied" as it might appear. The bulk of our intake nowadays consists of extensively purified carbohydrates, mainly starches and sugars—as well as substantial amounts of fats and oils. To a diner there is a big difference between a sweet roll and a bowl of presweetened cereal, but to the gastrointestinal system, they are nearly identical. Instant mashed potatoes seem quite a different dish from a plateful of white rice, but from a nutritional point of view they are almost identical.

The second question is: "How can a single deficiency be responsible for diseases as different from one another as heart attacks, cancer of the colon, diverticular disease of the colon, and hemorrhoids?"

The answer: Each of those conditions is directly related to the digestion and metabolism of food and the operation of the digestive system. As the story unfolds we will be able to consider the far-reaching evidence that conclusively proves this point. But first let's go back a century in time to examine the missing pieces in the dietary puzzle.

In the Western world about 1880 a strange obsession began to appear. For some years before that time men of wealth, aristocrats, and, of course, royalty had eaten nothing but white bread. The peasants and poor city dwellers were compelled to settle for "black" bread, which was made from coarsely milled flour. Presumably consumers rated their bread on a "prestige scale"—white bread was considered "pure" and dark bread, containing substantial amounts of roughage, was considered "impure."

In those days, the flour mills used stone grinding wheels, and since their surfaces were rough, no matter how well they were positioned, the wheat berries could not be smashed completely. Even carefully ground wheat flour still contained a fair amount of bran and other fiber. (Flour that was whitened by sifting through cloths was a high-cost item for the rich.)

But suddenly in the 1880's there was a revolution in the milling industry: the steel rolling mill was introduced. Since the precisely-polished steel surfaces mated perfectly, the grains of wheat could be smashed finer than ever before. That enabled millers to easily extract most of the fiber and produce a low-cost, high-prestige, nearly pure-white flour. The new roller mills also had an important incidental advantage. One of the annoyances of the flour trade was the relatively high loss of stored wheat to insects. But the ultra-refined flour had so much of the nutrient material removed that it was barely able to keep bugs alive—therefore insect infestation was reduced considerably. The irony of feeding men, women, and children with flour that couldn't keep bugs alive was lost on those early millers.

Those changes in milling practices were critical to the health of the average person, since in the nineteenth century an average person consumed about one pound of flour a day—mostly in the form of bread. These days the average person eats about six ounces of flour daily or less than half as much.

At the same time that most of the fiber was taken out of the flour, the consumption of sugar began to increase. Going back to 1815, the average Englishman consumed about ten pounds of sugar *a year*; his American cousin, somewhat less. By 1965 he was taking in *one hundred and twenty pounds* yearly, or his previous total annual consumption *every month*. Americans eat about 158 pounds of sugar a year or about their total body weight in sugar. One problem with sugar from the standpoint of the fiber-deficiency diseases is that it contains no fiber at all. At the same time, it is so filling that it cuts down the appetite for roughage-containing foods.

As time went by, more and more of the diet of Western man has come to consist of sugar in various forms combined with white-flour products and refined carbohydrates such as ultra-refined bread, cereals, doughnuts, cakes, pies, cookies, and white rice. There seem to have been some beneficial changes in the diet in that period—at least at first glance. The average consumption of fruit and vegetables in 1909 was about 146 pounds per person per year. By 1970 that had increased to 273 pounds yearly. Unfortunately much of the fiber content has been lost by peeling, boiling, canning, dehydrating, and otherwise processing that category of food. In addition, we tend to consume new strains of low-fiber fruits and vegetables adapted to modern taste—some examples being the "stringless" string bean and the "burp-less" cucumber.

To medical researchers, the mass of evidence now seemed to implicate the modern low-roughage diet as an important cause of the serious diseases of modern civilization. Nutritionists and scientists all over the world became more and more intrigued. But there was one important loophole in the evidence that needed to be plugged before the facts could be considered conclusive. If a deficiency of fiber or roughage was to be proved responsible for the massive increase in lethal and destructive diseases, then simply comparing the health of the rural Africans with the health of Western man was not enough. The ultimate confirmation would come if it were possible to show that as the dietary fiber was removed from the Western diet—as we ate less roughage—we began to succumb to these terrible afflictions. The search for that confirmatory evidence set off a minutely detailed examination of medical records around the world. Based on the fact that the substantial reduction of roughage in flour began about 1880, this is what the researchers found:

1. Heart attacks—which we accept as a daily occurrence—were *extremely rare in the United States and Britain until about the 1920's.* Then suddenly from 1931 to 1971 in England and Wales coronary heart disease—the cause of 'heart attacks'—increased *800 percent!*

2. Appendicitis—the disease that shows up some twenty to thirty years before the other, more deadly effects of a roughage-deficient diet, was very rare before 1880. Subsequently it became a very common and almost predictable event.

3. Diverticular disease of the colon only emerged as a common disease in the late 1920's. In Britain, between 1931 and 1971 the death rate from that condition increased *600 percent!*

4. Even obesity, which we take for granted as part of our modern way of life, was a disease that generally affected only the wealthy in eighteenth century Europe.

These are just a few of the most outstanding and dramatic examples. Painstaking review of the medical records reveals that the same general progression applies to each of the major conditions. There are millions of individual bits of evidence in scores of countries around the world that confirm and reconfirm the basic premise: ***As the amount of roughage in the diet decreases, the incidence of heart attacks, cancer of the colon and rectum, diverticulosis of the colon, and all the rest increase in almost direct proportion.*** In each case—except for the standard-bearer, appendicitis, which appears earlier—there seems to be a time lag of about fifty years— enough time for the body to lose its natural defenses and undergo a certain amount of deterioration in function.

By the time all this evidence was in, our modern fiber-deficient diet was almost unanimously indicted by international medical experts as the basic cause of these death-and-disability-dealing diseases.

To recapitulate, the chain of evidence was as follows:

1. These diseases are virtually unknown in individuals and cultures consuming a high-roughage diet.

2. They are catastrophically common in individuals and societies where the diet is low in roughage or dietary fiber.

3. When high-roughage individuals or groups switch to low-roughage diets, they gradually but relentlessly succumb to these diseases.

A close look at the typical American diet gives some idea of the extent of the hazard. Let's take three average American meals and rate them for their fiber and sugar content:

BREAKFAST:

Orange-flavored breakfast drink
White bread toasted with butter and jelly
Two eggs, any style
Coffee with sugar

LUNCH:

Sandwich with assorted luncheon meat on white bread
Soft drink
Lettuce salad

DINNER:

Roast beef, mashed potatoes, frozen peas
White bread
Ice cream

Three Meal Rating: High Refined Sugar ... Very Little Fiber.

If those three meals are consumed on *Monday*, the complete processing and digestion will be concluded, on the average, by late

Wednesday, and the residual material from the menu will be passed in a small, hard, constipated bowel movement *on **Friday** morning. If the same American family had consumed a readily-available high fiber diet on the same day, the food would have been completely processed by the next morning and all the residual products eliminated by Tuesday at the latest.* Ironically, the high-roughage diet (as we shall see) is more appetizing, less expensive, more satisfying, and more conducive to weight reduction than its low-roughage equivalent.

Even more tantalizing is the tiny amount of fiber that makes the difference between the possibility of cancer, heart attacks, and all the rest of the destructive diseases and the almost total immunity enjoyed by those on high-fiber diets.

On the average African villagers consume slightly less than *one ounce* (25 grams) of fiber per day. Modern Americans and Britons consume about *one-quarter ounce* of fiber daily (8 grams). The balance between potential health and potential disease is tipped by three-quarters of an ounce of almost indigestible fibrous material costing, at the most, two cents a day. *In a year, twelve pounds of roughage added to the average diet at a total cost of a little over seven dollars provides a million dollars worth of life and health insurance.*

Is there any risk involved in adding roughage to the usual roughage-deficient diet? It's hard to see what the risk might be, since we are only restoring the diet to what it was for the 50,000 years up to about 1880. Man, left to his own instinct, had naturally chosen a high-fiber non-fattening diet that encouraged the natural and normal functioning of his digestive system and protected him from the most horrendous diseases of "modern" civilization.

But to convict the fiber-deficient diet once and for all, one last loophole has to be closed. We need to demonstrate exactly how low-fiber diets do their terrible damage and show how high-fiber diets restore and maintain the body in a state of maximum health. The simplest and most objective way to judge the evidence is to examine what goes on in the human body day after day. Let's start at the beginning of the story—the digestive system.

3

How The Wrong Diet Can Cause Cancer Of The Colon And Rectum And Exactly How To Avoid It

The process of digestion is one of the true miracles of the universe. Everything an individual consumes passes through about forty feet of complicated gastrointestinal tubing and is acted upon by approximately two dozen chemical compounds. In the process such diverse dishes as frog's legs, calves' brains, oxtails, and pig's feet are converted to the basic building blocks of the human body.

Briefly, this is the way the process works:

Once the food is chewed and swallowed, it passes into the stomach, where it is mixed with hydrochloric acid and digestive chemicals. It then passes into the small intestine—twenty-three feet of relatively small-diameter flexible pipe. Secretions from the liver are added, via the gall bladder, and other enzymes are secreted by the pancreas. By this time the food is well mashed and uniformly mixed with the digestive chemicals. Although some absorption may have occurred in the stomach, the major part of the nutrition is extracted from the food in the small intestine. Then the mushy mass of almost totally digested food is pushed into the colon. As far as most students of nutrition are concerned, that's when the game is over. As far as we are concerned, that's when things really get interesting!

For all too many years the five or so feet of the large intestine or colon were considered to be the sewage disposal plant of the body. The colon was viewed as a sort of septic tank to hold fecal material between bowel movements. As a result of many years of ingenious and sophisticated research it has now become obvious that the colon plays a vital role in the destiny of the human organism.

Instead of a stagnant holding tank, the colon is actually a living river. The dregs of digestion (feces is the plural of the Latin word faex, which means "dregs") are half liquid and half solid, and flow through the colon like an active stream. The solid portion of the fecal material travels in front of the liquid part and the wall of the intestine selectively soaks up excess water.

For hundreds of years people have instinctively felt that there was something vaguely undesirable about allowing those dregs to accumulate day after day in that large flexible tube deep in the abdomen. Our grandparents prescribed "high enemas" or "colonic irrigations" to dispose of fecal accumulations. Even today there is a billion-dollar sale of laxatives designed to empty the colon of its contents. (An interesting fringe benefit of the extensive research on the effects of roughage showed the undesirability of taking laxatives for this purpose and even indicated that one type of commonly prescribed laxative can damage the nerves that control the large intestine.)

Without knowing why, our old-fashioned forebears were on the right track. One of the greatest risks a human being can take is to allow the remnants of his food—that is, the fecal end products— to remain in contact with the lining of his colon for three and four days at a time. And that's exactly what 99 percent of Americans and others who eat a "modern" diet are doing. At the end of their digestive tract they are harboring a time bomb. This is what the researchers in laboratories around the world found:

Every cancer researcher agrees that cancer can be caused by body surfaces coming in contact with potent cancer-causing chemicals known as carcinogens. Unfortunately, there are examples all around us. Vinyl chloride as a cause of fatal cancer of the liver has gotten a great deal of publicity lately. Many of the food additives that have recently been banned are known or suspected to have caused cancer in human beings. The actual list of cancer-producing chemicals contains many hundreds of items, most of them organic chemicals with exotic names like methyl cholanthrene and the like.

In the process of studying cancer of the colon in rats, (animals that have a body metabolism much like humans) one investigator made a startling discovery. He fed a drug called cycasin to a group of normal rats. As expected, many of them promptly developed cancer of the colon.

Then, on impulse, he tried the same experiment with a group of special rats who had been raised in such a way that their bodies were absolutely free of bacteria. To his amazement, none of the bacteria-free rats developed cancer. He then went on to analyze the urine and feces from both groups of rats, and what he found has life-and-death implications for over three hundred million Americans. In the germ-free—and thus cancer-free—rats, the cancer-producing drug cycasin was recovered unchanged in the urine and feces. But in the cancer-ridden rats, only 35 percent of the chemical, at the most, was found in those waste products. That meant that the bacteria in the colon of the cancerous rats had broken down the cycasin into powerful, cancer-causing chemicals!

Turning their attention to human beings, scientists made a parallel and even more astonishing discovery. The human liver normally produces a chemical cocktail which we call bile. It is a thick greenish liquid essential for digestion, especially for the breakdown of fats. Bile is composed of several different chemicals known as bile acids that go by such arcane names as cholic acid and deoxycholic acid. (Incidentally, it is the pigments of bile that give feces their brownish color. If for some reason the liver is obstructed, as in hepatitis, bile cannot enter the small intestine and the bowel movement becomes pale, almost white, in color. The pigment may find its way into the skin and turn it greenish-yellow, causing jaundice.)

In any event, the investigators found that the average low-roughage-consuming American has two nutritionally significant types of bacteria in his colon; the dominant groups are known as bacteroides and bifidobacteria. It has been proved beyond any doubt that the common bile acid, cholic acid, can be converted into the powerful cancer-causing chemical, apcholic acid *by these bacteria.*

Likewise the other bile acid, deoxycholic acid, can be changed into one of the most deadly of all known carcinogens, 3-methyl-cholanthrene.

The implications of those discoveries are simple and unequivocal: Americans who are on lifelong low-roughage diets are converting their own harmless bile acids into awesome cancer-producing compounds deep within the dark chambers of their own large intestines!

Further proof lies in the fact that individuals on low-roughage diets pass decreased amounts of bile acids in their bowel movements, indicating that, like cancerous rats, they have broken them down into cancer-causing compounds.

On the other hand, people who consume high-roughage diets have a colon dominated by streptococcus and lactobacillus bacteria, which do not to attack bile acids and break them down. As additional confirmation of this protection, high-roughage individuals pass a much greater proportion of intact, unchanged bile acids in their feces.

Assuming that these potentially lethal chemicals are accumulating in the colon as each day passes, the body's next line of defense is to get them out of contact with the soft and vulnerable lining of the large intestine. Ironically, only those on high-roughage diets—who are never exposed to the cancer chemicals—don't have to worry on that score. They store their freshest fecal products in the colon for less than eighteen hours on the average, based on the fact that experimental time-markers pass through their entire digestive tracts in about twenty-four hours.

The low-roughage cancer-producing American diet allows the fecal mass and its store of cancer chemicals to wash over the colon for seventy-two hours or longer—and in the case of some British patients, for as long as two weeks. Even our valuable and dedicated astronauts are deliberately fed a special low-roughage diet which delays their bowel movements as long as six days. Beyond that, each bowel movement consists of 20 to 30 percent bacteria—so the faster any bile-acid-splitting bacteria are moved out of the intestine, the less mischief they can perform.

Other experiments leave little doubt that encouraging prolonged contact between the remnants of digestion and the wall of the colon is inviting disaster. In those experimental animals that are deliberately given cancer, simply isolating loop of intestine so that feces never flow over it prevents malignant changes in that isolated loop. There is a further fascinating observation made by a leading researcher:

For all practical purposes, only two epithelial-lined body channels are common sites of cancer—the bronchial tubes, which are the location of the most common form of lung cancer, and the colon. These are—not by coincidence—the only channels or tubes that are exposed to foreign substances. The bronchial tubes are exposed to cigarette smoke and the colon is exposed to the slow-moving fecal stream containing residual cancer-causing chemicals from unnaturally low-roughage foods.

The irony of being an unwilling accomplice in the development of one's own colon cancer is compounded by the fact that modern therapy for cancer of the colon is not really encouraging. In fact, it has not basically changed since 1900. The strategy is to wait helplessly until the cancer is firmly established within your large intestine. As the cancer grows, you have pain, bleeding, diarrhea, or constipation. Then, as the cancer is enlarging day by day, medical science finally makes a dedicated and valiant effort to save your life.

The actual treatment of the malignant tumor is based on destroying the affected part of the organ as well as a sizable amount of healthy tissue. In many cases of cancer of the colon and the extension of the colon, the rectum, that means closing off the anus and repositioning it permanently in the abdominal wall. (The feces then are caught in a plastic bag glued to the patient's abdomen.) In some cases, tumor tissue (and an unavoidable amount of normal tissue) is destroyed by radiation—similar to the fallout from a nuclear explosion. Patients are also treated on occasion by chemotherapy— that is, the administration of extremely toxic drugs designed to kill tumor cells without excessively-damaging the patient's body permanently. Tragically, in spite of the Herculean efforts of devoted specialists, about half of those stricken with colon cancer don't survive and for some types of colon cancer the survival rate is even declining! How much better it would be to simply add roughage to one's diet and drastically reduce the risk of ever succumbing to colon cancer.

Unfortunately, the risk for Americans is a very real one. The United States has nearly the highest rate of colon cancer in the world.

About 54 out of every 100,000 American men develop cancer of the colon or rectum. It seems more than a coincidence that our national diet is nearly the lowest in roughage of any nation in the world. By contrast, the incidence of colon cancer in the United States is 900 percent greater than that of Nigeria and 1,300 percent greater than Uganda, two countries with traditional high-roughage diets.

Although rural black Africans are protected from cancer of the colon by their high-roughage diet, that immunity does not extend to their American cousins. After two generations of living in the United States and gradually shifting to a low-fiber diet, the rate for colon cancer among African-Americans is almost identical to that of their Caucasian fellow citizens. That's exactly what one would expect, since both African-Americans and Caucasian digestive systems now operate in deadly slow motion. The same misfortune has befallen second-generation Japanese who have moved to Hawaii and forsaken the traditional Japanese high-fiber diet. The rate of colon malignancy is also rising among those who dwell in Japan but have made the transition to low-roughage foods.

As far as cancer of the colon is concerned, it seems that more than enough evidence is in to convict the modern low-fiber diet.

That's the bad news. But the good news is that cancer of the colon—and rectum—is a potentially preventable disease. And the most likely way to prevent it is simply to restore the human diet to what it should be and to what it used to be before cancer of the large intestine killed and crippled so many victims every year. Remember, the longer we delay changing our diet the greater the chances that it will be too late.

The same holds true—perhaps even more urgently—when it comes to heart attacks.

4

How The Wrong Diet Can Cause A Heart Attack And Exactly How To Avoid It

The average American male over the age of forty is living on borrowed time. According to the latest medical statistics, he has one chance out of two suffering a heart attack sometime before his sixty-fifth birthday. When that day comes, it will probably happen like this:

One summery Saturday afternoon after mowing the lawn, he will be slumped in his easy chair watching television and munching a snack. Without any warning he will suddenly feel a massive crushing pain just over his breastbone, "as if an elephant is sitting on his chest." He will instantly break out in a cold sweat and experience that indescribably agonizing feeling that doctors call *angor animi*—the sudden and chilling awareness that death is *imminent*.

If he is lucky—and that's the scientifically accurate word—he will be rushed to the hospital in an ambulance, hooked up to a collection of shiny electronic gadgets, given oxygen, various medications, and other emergency treatment. A few weeks later he will leave the hospital with one-tenth to one-third of his heart muscle *totally and permanently destroyed*. And that's what happens if he's *lucky*.

If he's *unlucky*, before the ambulance arrives he will slip into shock, the delicate electric circuits within the heart that control the heartbeat will be severely damaged, his heart rate will zoom to over three hundred beats a minute—and before they run the six o'clock news, he will be *dead*.

Many heart victims fall between these two extremes— some linger a few days or weeks in the hospital before slipping away. Others survive the attack but become cardiac cripples because of recurring chest pain or because not enough heart muscle has survived to efficiently pump blood through the body.

The actual figures are far from encouraging: only about 60 percent of all heart-attack victims survive the first attack (six-week survival rate), and the typical life expectancy of those who recover is only *five to seven years*. Yet the vast majority of heart attacks *never have to happen*. The tragedy that accounts for *one-third of all the deaths in the United States each year* is virtually unknown among *billions* of men and women in other parts of the world. It isn't the fast-paced life of modern society that causes those deadly heart attacks. Sudden agonizing death or lifelong disability doesn't have to be the price of success.

The *basic* difference between those who are nearly immune to heart attacks and those more than *one million three hundred thousand* Americans who annually suffer heart attacks is basically a matter of diet. A simple, appetizing, and cheap addition to the deadly American diet can provide *more efficient protection from heart attacks than any other means known to medical science*.

First, consider a few simple facts about the human heart. Basically the heart is nothing more than a hollow muscle that works like a simple pump—it squeezes blood through the body by contracting and relaxing about seventy times a minute. If you take a rubber ball in your hand and squeeze it, then allow it to snap back, you will very nearly duplicate the action of your own heart.

Of course, there are some important differences. Your hand gets tired after about a dozen squeezes, but your heart must *never* get tired. If you live to the age of seventy-five, your heart muscle will contract and relax about forty-seven million times— hopefully without missing a beat. That means 657,000 hours of nonstop functioning. If you give it a chance, your heart can do it—it has ample capacity to spare.

In those few persons who live to the age of a hundred and twenty, the heart beats *seventy-five million* times. But there is one indispensable requirement: that tough little heart muscle must have a constant and adequate supply of oxygen. The heart actually provides its own blood and oxygen requirements via the coronary arteries—a system of tiny blood vessels that circle the cardiac muscle. If, without warning, one day these miniature arteries that supply blood to the heart become obstructed, the nightmare of a heart attack becomes a sudden catastrophic reality.

All it takes is a tiny blood clot to clog the delicate tubing—which is no larger in diameter than a pencil lead. Then, as the heart muscle is deprived of life-giving oxygen, it slowly sickens and dies. Obstruction of the blood supply to the heart impairs the ability of that muscle to pump blood to the rest of the body *and to itself*. As it continues to fail, it progressively reduces its own source of oxygen and fails even more rapidly.

Then the complex electrical pacemaker buried deep in the wall of the heart muscle starts to fail and the precisely-controlled muscular contractions of this marvel-of-engineering become irregular and haphazard. The stage is set for the ultimate catastrophe—cardiac *shock* and cardiac *death*. But even if the individual survives, there is one immense problem. Heart muscle is different from any other type of muscle in the body—especially in one unfortunate way. *It does not regenerate*. Once a portion of the heart dies, it stays dead, and the burden of contracting 103,000 times a day to pump the blood has to be borne by whatever tattered remnant of the cardiac muscle survives.

Yet heart attacks can be prevented. By combining the insights of scientists and researchers around the world, it is finally possible for potential victims to provide themselves with more protection against heart attacks—with less risk—than ever before.

Part of that protection hinges on understanding why that blood clot obstructs the tiny coronary artery in the first place. Most expert cardiologists agree that cholesterol is the primary cause of heart attacks. This greasy substance gradually accumulates in arteries of the human body over a period of years. It functions much like corrosion in household plumbing—clinging to the walls of the blood vessels, roughening their surfaces, and slowly narrowing their diameters. (Often the body deposits rock-like calcium into the cholesterol corrosion, adding to the problem.) Finally the tragic day comes when the tiny arteries to the heart are made so narrow by cholesterol deposits that the flow of blood begins to slow. Then a tiny clot can form, and what started out as a lazy Saturday afternoon turns into the ordeal of a lifetime.

By eliminating cholesterol from the body we should be able to eliminate all risk of heart attacks. There's only one problem: cholesterol gets into the bloodstream and the arteries in two ways. First, it is consumed in a wide variety of foods including most animal fats or animal fat-containing substances. The list includes butter, eggs, lard, whole milk, cheese, cream, and meat. Even if it were possible to eliminate all these appetizing items from the menu, it wouldn't affect the second source of cholesterol: the body itself.

The human liver synthesizes cholesterol in impressive amounts, and there are even some experts who feel that cutting down on the amount of cholesterol in the diet, forces the liver to produce more cholesterol within the body. In any event, cholesterol is not harmful in itself—as a matter of fact, it is essential for the normal functioning of the human body. However, when the amount of cholesterol circulating in the blood rises above, say, 300 milligrams in each 100 milliliters of blood—known as "300 milligrams percent" or "300 mg %"—the chances for a heart attack *increase* dramatically. Doctors have proved over and over again that reducing the cholesterol in the blood to normal levels—about 200 mg % or less—substantially *reduces* the chance of a heart attack.

There are two safe practical ways to reduce the blood level of cholesterol. The first way is the simplest and most obvious: merely reduce the amount of fatty, cholesterol-rich foods that you eat. That involves concentrating on items which are high in what is called "unsaturated fats"—like corn oil and safflower oil—and restricting the intake of meat, eggs, cheese, and milk.

Unfortunately, abandoning the eating habits of a lifetime isn't an easy task—and to be honest, a low-fat diet involves a lot of sacrifice for the ones who eat it and the ones who cook it. The menu must be reworked to avoid or minimize eggs, bacon, butter, most cooking oils (except unsaturated ones like safflower and corn oils and the like), most forms of cheese, many kinds of shellfish, whole milk, ice cream, and the kind and quantity of meat that most people are used to eating. To further complicate the situation, the low-fat diet tends to be much more expensive than the ordinary American diet.

Beyond that, many convenience and commercial foods containing fat are prepared with low-cost fats, such as coconut oil or lard. These are precisely the saturated fats that must be banished from the menus of those on a low-fat anti-cholesterol diet. That puts many "instant" foods on the forbidden list and eliminates a lot of commercial bakery goods such as doughnuts, cream pies, cakes with icing, custards, and puddings.

But for those who are willing to make the sacrifices—both financially and in taste appeal—there is no doubt that the low-fat diet does reduce the cholesterol level somewhat. More important, massive and costly studies of large groups of men have proven that a low-fat diet statistically reduces the chances of a heart attack. In spite of whatever advantages it may have, the standard low-fat diet is also a *low-roughage diet* with all its potential for triggering that terrifying form of lethal cancer, cancer of the colon and rectum.

By one of those happy coincidences that occur so rarely in the world of science, the same diet that protects against colon cancer can also effectively lower blood cholesterol and give dramatic protection from heart attacks. Consuming a diet high in cereal fiber—that is, a high-roughage diet—has been *incontrovertibly proven to increase the excretion of cholesterol from the body.* In fact, a high-roughage diet gives the best of both worlds. It increases the amount of cholesterol that is excreted in the daily bowel movement at the same time it reduces the amount of cholesterol secreted by the liver. Let's see how the process works.

A certain amount of the cholesterol normally produced by the liver is converted by the body into bile acids—the same substances we saw in the explanation of cancer of the colon. These bile acids ultimately find their way to the colon, where they are vulnerable to destruction by the massive number of bacteria which are present. Those individuals who consume low-roughage diets—that is, most Americans—harbor billions of anti-bile acid bacteria in their colons. These immediately act to break down the bile acids into two important types of substances (among others)—a group of cancer-causing chemicals and a toxic substance called "lithocholate."

Lithocholate specifically acts back on the liver to cut down the conversion of cholesterol into bile acids.

That results in two unfortunate consequences. First, as less cholesterol is broken down into bile acids, cholesterol tends to accumulate in the bloodstream—*and in the arteries to the heart*. Secondly, *less cholesterol finds its way into the colon*—in the form of bile acids—where it can be excreted in the feces. That is extremely critical since *the major pathway for ridding the body of hazardous and unwanted cholesterol is via the colon and the bowel movement*. There is no doubt about this mechanism since it has been proved thousands of times in man and experimental animals.

A high-roughage diet seems to alter the type of bacteria that dominate the colon. Thus when the bile acids arrive from the liver they are greeted by the friendly high-roughage-produced bacteria and are rapidly excreted in the bowel movement almost intact. That not only gets rid of significant amounts of cholesterol each day, but in a sense tricks the liver into "wasting" more and more cholesterol by converting it into bile acids that are soon eliminated. It is a beautiful, elegant, and natural way of protecting the body against one of its worst internal enemies, excessive cholesterol, and there is no doubt that it works.

In a study performed in Holland, volunteers on a diet containing rolled oats—high in roughage—brought their cholesterol down from an average of 251 mg % to 223 mg %, *in only twenty-one days*. That is particularly impressive since they started at a level lower than that of most middle-aged overweight Americans. Predictably, when they resumed a conventional *low-roughage* diet, their cholesterol zoomed to its previous level within three weeks.

Even more amazing, high-roughage diets produce lower cholesterol levels *even though the subject may continue to eat a high-fat diet*. First observed in animals, that important finding was confirmed in a project involving two matched groups of men. One group consumed a high-fat diet plus low roughage. The other group also ate a high-fat diet but consumed an adequate amount of roughage. The high-fat, low-roughage men had cholesterol levels of 206 mg % while the high-fat, high-roughage group had cholesterol readings of 160mg percent—a difference of *22 percent*. Even more convincing, those on a low-roughage diet excreted a mere 236 milligrams of dangerous bile acids a day, while those eating enough substantial fiber got rid of 305 milligrams of dangerous bile acids daily—almost *30 percent more.*

To summarize, these facts seem well-documented:

1. The basic cause of heart attacks is large amounts of cholesterol circulating in the bloodstream and being deposited in the arteries of the heart.

2. A. high-roughage diet reduces the absolute amount of cholesterol in the bloodstream in two ways:

(a) by forcing the liver to convert cholesterol into bile salts, and subsequently,

(b) increasing the amount of bile salts that are passed in the bowel movement.

So the solution to high blood cholesterol levels—and the resulting massive death rate from heart attacks—may be a happy one. It is just possible that once they restore the roughage to their diet, Americans can continue eating pretty much what they have been eating as their doctors watch their cholesterol levels descend to normal.

It seems likely that the real problem of elevated blood cholesterol—and the resultant heart attacks—may not depend so much on the type and amount of fat which you consume. The most vital factor—and the difference between life and death for millions of Americans—may be the massive amounts of cholesterol that their livers are compelled to pour out because of unending stimulation from decomposing bile acids deep within the darkest recesses of their colons. It may well be that increasing the roughage in your diet—and thereby keeping the bile acids intact—will allow the wisdom of your own body to protect you from the needless tragedy and suffering of our society's great destroyer, the heart attack.

5

Diverticulosis And Appendicitis: The Treatment Can Make You Sicker

Diverticulosis is the single most common disease of the colon. Approximately 40 percent of all Americans over the age of forty are its victims and almost 70 percent of those past seventy years old suffer from the disease.

It has reached endemic proportions in North America and Europe and causes untold suffering and disability. The most astounding aspect of the condition is that as recently as 1916 it was so rare that it was not even mentioned in medical textbooks! Like some strange new island arising from the depths of the ocean, diverticulosis has suddenly appeared to blight the lives of millions. Even in 1960 official medical opinion held that diverticulosis was a "symptomless disease," a "silent benign condition". It is now well-established as a cause of the following collection of symptoms:

1. Nausea
2. Heartburn
3. Excessive gas
4. Bloating and distention
5. Severe abdominal pain
6. Rectal tenderness
7. Incomplete emptying of the rectum
8. Constipation

No one knows exactly how many millions of Americans suffer from diverticulosis because many cases are never even diagnosed while the patient is still alive. The victims waste tens of millions of dollars each year on antacid pills, powders, and liquids which generally provide little relief of the symptoms and allow the disease to progress.

Unfortunately, that's the least of it. Almost two out of every ten cases of diverticulosis progress to *diverticulitis*, a dangerous and potentially fatal disease that can involve constant pain, chills, fever, bleeding, and ultimately perforation of the intestine and ... *death*.

Let's take a moment to look at the design and function of the colon so that we can understand exactly what diverticulosis and diverticulitis are, what causes them, and how they can be prevented or cured.

The human large intestine, or colon, can be compared to a long string of joined very short link sausages. At the point where each sausage is joined together at the end, the colon has a circular band of muscle which can expand and contract. In effect, these muscular bands function as valves at the end of each segment, opening and closing in perfect synchronization to move the intestinal contents forward on their way out of the body. As one end of a segment opens, the other end closes, the muscles contract and the feces move ahead. The effect is like that of a digestive conveyor belt pushing the semiliquid feces forward progressively. If all goes well, the feces are hustled out of the body in short order. Success in this conveying project depends on three elements:

1. Maintaining the diameter of the colon as wide as possible—the larger the pipe, the faster the flow.

2. Assuring that the contents are liquid or at least semiliquid to avoid allowing too much water to be absorbed from the feces and drying the fecal mass.

3. Being sure to empty the fecal contents promptly when the urge arises to prevent further drying and hardening.

But if all doesn't go well, things turn out quite differently. If the products of digestion drift lazily through the colon, as the months and years go by the diameter of the colon shrinks down. That obviously lengthens transport time, since a one-inch pipe cannot provide the flow that a four-inch pipe can. Meanwhile, water is continuously being absorbed from the fecal material, which becomes progressively harder and drier. These factors cause a critical increase in the internal pressure in the colon—and that's where big problems start.

The wall of the colon isn't very strong to begin with, and at its weakest points it begins to bulge out in a series of blisters like tiny rubber balloons. Once the thin stretchy wall of the colon pops out in these bubbles, *it never goes back to normal.* Instead of a large-bore smooth-walled colon, the unfortunate victim of diverticulosis is left with a narrow pipe that has many pockets and bulges along its length. Digestion is profoundly disturbed and the eight major symptoms of diverticular disease may suddenly become prominent:

1. Nausea

2. Heartburn

3. Excessive gas

4. Bloating and distention

5. Severe abdominal pain

6. Rectal tenderness

7. Incomplete emptying of the rectum

8. Constipation

The diagnosis is easily made by taking an X-ray of the large intestine—one or dozens of the little pouches are clearly seen protruding from the sides of the colon. Sometimes a small piece of hardened fecal matter can plug up the narrow neck of these balloons (or "diverticula," as they are known)—or the opening that connects the pouch with the colon can become obstructed on its own. Then inflammation, infection, and abscess formation can occur. When that happens, *diverticulosis* gives way to *diverticulitis*—the "-itis" ending on the word signifies that *infection* of those little balloons is the problem. Severe pain, massive bleeding, and even death can occur as a result.

From about 1920—when diverticulosis and diverticulitis were first recognized as distinct diseases—until recently, the treatment was, to say the least, unexciting. The usual therapy for diverticulosis was mineral oil as a laxative to combat the stubborn constipation and a *low-roughage diet,* supposedly to "rest" the colon. In some cases, even surgery was performed. For diverticulitis, the treatment was morphine for pain, antibiotics and rest for the infection, and for severe cases *surgical removal* of the affected part of the intestine. The patients weren't satisfied because their suffering usually went on unabated. The physicians weren't satisfied because they were neither able to understand nor effectively treat the most widely encountered disease of the colon.

Then, fortunately for all of us, the same group of British (and later American) physicians and surgeons who pioneered in the discovery of high-roughage diets as the prevention of colon cancer, heart attacks, and other conditions turned their attention to diverticulosis and diverticulitis. Even in the early stages of their investigation they were struck by some fascinating findings.

First, they observed that diverticulosis and diverticulitis were extremely rare in Africa, Korea, Singapore, Malaysia, Iran, India, New Guinea and other areas depending on a high-roughage diet. Conversely, the diseases were very common in areas of low-roughage consumption such as the United States and Britain.

Predictably, the incidence was intermediate in countries where the diet was in transition from high roughage to low roughage. Further evidence came from the fact that during World War II the incidence of diverticulosis actually *decreased* in Britain when the only available bread had a much higher roughage content—and, incidentally, where ultra-refined carbohydrates like sugar were in very short supply. Elsewhere in the world the researchers discovered that those who were in the process of switching from a high-roughage diet to a low-roughage diet faced mounting affliction with diverticular disease. That included the Hawaiian and Californian Japanese, Afro-Americans, and city-dwelling Africans. Additional confirmation of the role that low-roughage diets played in diverticulosis came from the fact that those who succumbed to the other diseases of low-roughage diet intake—such as heart attacks, appendicitis, hemorrhoids, and cancer of the colon—also had a higher-than-average incidence of diverticular disease. *Even rats maintained on a low-roughage diet came down with diverticulosis.*

The next step was a bold one. A few intrepid physicians abandoned the traditional low-roughage diet and deliberately fed *high-roughage* diets to diverticulosis patients. That set off a firestorm of criticism. They were accused of irritating the already hyper-irritable intestine by forcing it to deal with the seeds, strings, and skins contained in vegetables and subjecting the intestine to even larger amounts of cereal fiber. *But the results proved the doctors right.*

In one pioneer study carried out in England, seventy patients who had received little benefit from the traditional low-roughage treatment were exposed to the high-roughage diet. *Sixty-two out of seventy obtained dramatic relief.* That translates into a relief rate of about *88 percent—without* drugs, *without* surgery, and *without* risk. Nearly all of them were able to discontinue their previous medications and lead a normal life.

The same kind of results were obtained over and over again in subsequent groups of patients until, at the present time, more and more physicians are selecting a high-roughage diet as *the standard treatment* for diverticulosis. Interestingly enough, once it absorbs water and is processed by the digestive system, "roughage" quickly becomes "softage" and rapidly restores the way the intestine works to normal.

Regrettably no amount of dietary alteration can restore the *structure* of the ballooned-out portions of the colon to normal, although as long as patients remain on their high-fiber diet, they are remarkably free of symptoms.

There is one vitally important lesson to be learned from the experience with diverticulosis. Since the disease apparently takes about forty years or so to damage the intestinal wall, the ideal time to begin avoiding the irreversible damage is during childhood. A child who is raised on the typical American high-sugar, ultra-refined carbohydrate, low-roughage diet has every chance of developing serious diverticular disease—not to mention cancer of the colon, heart attacks, and all the rest.

The major offenders in the average child's diet are:

1. White bread

2. Low-roughage sugar-strewn breakfast cereals

3. High-sugar soft drinks

4. Hamburgers, pizzas, hot dogs, ice cream, and low-fiber dessert products including those aimed specifically at children.

Ironically, with about the same effort, the same manufacturers can produce high-quality high-roughage products with a better taste and greater nutritional value. To make matters worse, some cereal manufacturers actually make high-roughage products but deliberately do not promote them to children or parents. Most of these high-fiber type cereals are aimed at older folks where much of the damage has already been done.

Another consequence of the traditional low-roughage diet is particularly unfortunate for youngsters and people under forty. That's the problem of appendicitis. Most of us consider inflammation of the appendix a relatively minor matter in comparison with cancer and heart disease. In the United States, however, appendicitis is the *number one abdominal emergency*—surgeons perform approximately *three hundred thousand appendectomies* each *year.* At an average cost of about $30,000, that adds up to the colossal cost of **9 billion dollars each year!** Much more tragic, there are about 389 deaths annually from appendicitis or its complications. That is intolerable—especially from a condition that is preventable and need never have happened in the first place. A brief survey of appendicitis brings the entire picture quickly into focus.

The full medical name of that little intestinal troublemaker is the "vermiform appendix"—that means "the wormlike tubing that hangs down." That's a pretty good description of the diminutive organ. About two and a half inches long, more or less the diameter of your little finger, the appendix is a short length of dead-end hollow tubing that leads off from the point where the small intestine goes into the large intestine. Anatomically, it usually lies just underneath a point several inches to the right and below your belt buckle. Its purpose has long since been forgotten—the appendix may be the remnant of a now-extinct extra length of intestinal tubing. Or—it may be useful protection against cancer and viruses. Many scientific studies have indicated that people who have appendectomies *develop cancer more often than those who preserve the original organ!* But one thing is certain— appendicitis or inflammation of the appendix is potentially dangerous. When appendicitis occurs, this is how it can happen:

At any hour of the day or night, without any warning whatsoever, the appendix swells and becomes inflamed. The tiny opening to the rest of the intestine is swiftly sealed, the little appendix is sealed off from the main part of the intestine and quickly fills with fluid. It then becomes hot, red, and infected and unless surgery is performed *immediately*, it may rupture.

When that happens, liquid feces are sprayed all over the abdominal cavity, resulting in potentially fatal peritonitis. One of the worst features of acute appendicitis is that it can happen anywhere and anytime. It is a death-dealing possibility in a spaceship on the way to the moon, in a submarine on the bottom of the ocean, in the Amazon jungle, and in the desolation of Antarctica. Less dramatically but more commonly, it can threaten mother and child during the course of a pregnancy.

A careful survey of incidence and extent of appendicitis reveals the same fascinating progression as the other low-roughage diseases—colon cancer, heart attacks, and all the rest. Before about 1880 appendicitis was a rare condition. Then slowly it began to crop up in Britain and the United States. About 1920 a distinguished English physician made the astute observation that appendicitis was frequent in affluent schoolboys who attended posh private schools and dined on low-fiber white bread, cakes, and pastry. It was much rarer in "unfortunate" orphans who subsisted on the cheap, coarse, high-fiber bread offered by the orphanage.

Later, investigators turned their attention to the underdeveloped countries and found what is by now a familiar pattern. Appendicitis was virtually unknown among those who followed a local high-roughage diet.

In one section of Africa, less than *3 percent* of the abdominal surgery performed on *Africans* was for appendicitis. In the same area, more than *30 percent* of the abdominal surgery performed on *Europeans* was for appendicitis. The major difference between the two groups was the amount of roughage in their respective diets.

In nation after nation, appendicitis was found to be a rare disease. In Kenya, Uganda, the Sudan, Ghana, Nigeria, Rhodesia, South Africa, Rumania, Egypt, and India, those on high-roughage diets hardly had to worry about inflammation of the appendix. Foreigners on low-roughage diets had the usual Western incidence of the disease.

In the process of the research there were some ingenious observations. For example, black African stevedores who worked unloading ships in the harbor seemed to have a higher rate of appendicitis than other members of their families. This apparent contradiction was finally explained when observers noted that the stevedores were fed on Western low-roughage fare from the ships they were unloading. Similarly, Sudanese soldiers who served in the British Army during World War II and Congolese students in Belgium all showed much higher rates of appendicitis than their relatives back home.

Further confirmation of the relation of diet to appendicitis was reaffirmed as the rate of appendicitis dropped in Switzerland during World War II when the Swiss ate less refined bread, more vegetables, and cut their consumption of refined carbohydrates such as sugar.

The exact mechanism that causes appendicitis is unclear, but it might well be this: Under the influence of a low-roughage diet, the entire digestive system goes into slow motion. The food dawdles on its way through the intestine, and as each hour passes, more and more of the water is absorbed. This encourages the formation of "fecaliths"—tiny, rock-hard pebbles of fecal material. As the fecal stream flows slowly through the intestines, one of these small concretions may drop into the opening to the appendix – like a golf ball dropping into a hole—and seal it off. The stagnant intestine may then allow bacteria to multiply and the resulting inflammation closes off the connection of the appendix to the intestine. The pressure within the appendix increases, stretching its already thin wall and making it vulnerable to the ever-present bacteria. Infection and inflammation soon follow and another red-hot appendix cries out for the surgeon's knife.

It does not seem to be a coincidence that those individuals who have had appendicitis also have an increased tendency to later develop cancer of the colon. It is probably another unfortunate legacy of the low-roughage diet.

As far as appendicitis is concerned, the chain of evidence is unbroken. Based on studies on the clinical course and medical records of millions of cases in over twenty countries during the past fifty years, *it seems obvious that appendicitis is a preventable disease.* Most of the 9 billion dollars stolen from our national economy each year and the lives wasted can probably be saved. All we have to do is restore the roughage to our diet—the same roughage that was there since the days of the cave men … until we took it out.

6

Constipation, Hemorrhoids, Varicose Veins, And Deadly Phlebitis, Four Accidents That Never Had To Happen

Constipation has the dual distinction of simultaneously being the most common and the most neglected affliction of modern times. In Western countries, nearly 100 percent of the population suffers from the condition at one time or another. Yet no one except the victims seems to take it seriously. Even the most prestigious medical books underestimate the importance of the malfunction:

"The physician must patiently explain that daily bowel movements are not essential, that no real harm comes from the bowel not moving for up to four days."

This text continues:

"A real ill often develops ... based on the fatuous conviction that the body must rid itself of fecal residues in a stereotyped way and very frequently."

On the other hand, almost everyone *instinctively* feels that their body functions best if they *do* have a regular, well-formed bowel movement every day without straining. Recently more and more evidence has accumulated to suggest that instinct is correct. Careful observations of groups in underdeveloped countries consuming unprocessed diets show that normal bowel patterns consist of daily bowel movements.

Regular bowel function seems rational from another point of view—we consume food daily, we digest food daily, and we should be able to eliminate residues of digestion daily. The human colon is not a stainless-steel holding tank; it is a living part of an organism which is continually absorbing a wide variety of potent chemicals from the feces it contains. The longer the feces remain putrefying in the colon, the greater the chance that serious consequences will occur. (As we have seen, cancer is a real danger; furthermore the chemicals produced in stagnant feces tend to increase blood cholesterol.)

Constipation, the production of dry hard stools at less than daily intervals, keeps the hazardous substances in the feces in intimate contact with the intestinal wall far longer than necessary. A man weighing one hundred eighty pounds who consumes a low-roughage diet might pass about one-quarter pound of feces daily. At that rate, it will take him about two years for his bowel movements to equal his body weight. By comparison, the same man on a high roughage diet might have a half-pound bowel movement daily and excrete his total body weight in a single year. That extra forty-four pounds of fecal residue which lies stagnant in his body for up to twelve months certainly can't do him any good.

If scientific medicine doesn't take constipation seriously, there are dozens of drug companies who do. They turn out a dazzling variety of powders, pills, liquids, and even candy and chewing gum, to do for people what they can't do for themselves. In the United States alone, the laxative industry garners millions and millions of dollars each year—and the products it purveys range all the way from harmless to hazardous. For example, mineral oil, a popular home laxative, can interfere with the absorption of vitamin A. And excessive use of certain laxatives has been shown to seriously damage the nerve network of portions of the colon. Continuous use of any laxative drug, of course, can interfere with the normal functioning of the digestive system and produce problems including a dependence on laxatives. Just as important, so much of the money spent on laxative preparations is money wasted. *Constipation is virtually impossible on a diet that contains adequate roughage.* The same two cents a day that buys protection from so many serious diseases also purchases freedom from constipation.

This is the way the process works: Dietary fiber is made up of three basic compounds—*lignin,* cellulose, and hemi-cellulose. If there is enough fiber in the diet these substances work in unison on the intestines to produce regular, easy-to-pass bowel movements.

The precise action of the three components of fiber against constipation as delineated by some researchers is a fascinating one. As the bacteria in the colon act on dietary fiber, one of the by-products they produce is a group of "fatty acids." These substances which go by names like acetic, butyric, and propionic acid—are natural laxatives, and on a high-roughage diet they guarantee regular evacuation of the fast-moving fecal contents.

At the same time one of the three components of roughage, lignin, seems to balance the laxative effects of dietary fiber and prevent runaway diarrhea. Roughage also works against constipation in two other ways. First, it increases the bulk of the bowel movement so that the fecal contents stimulate muscular action of the bowel and push their way through. Part of this is explained by the ability of each gram of fiber to increase the volume of the stool up to twenty times. Fiber also absorbs substantial amounts of water and may soak up additional liquid compounds from the small intestine.

The precise method of using roughage to overcome constipation is simple and straightforward.

High-Rough-age Diet Plan Number Three (see **Chapter 7**) *should provide prompt and permanent relief in nearly every case.* In one research project in Britain, nearly every patient was cured of constipation in short order by adding about half an ounce (fifteen grams) of bran to his daily diet. To make the daily roughage replacement even more appetizing—and incidentally more portable for those who must travel or eat in restaurants—another British team suggested a type of cracker which incorporates the total twenty-four-hour roughage requirement in a simple and appetizing form.

These crackers have been adapted to American tastes and the recipe appears in **Chapter 10** under the name "Hi-Fiber Crackers." Each of these tiny crisp onion, cheese, or garlic-flavored crackers contains about three grams of unprocessed bran; five of them provide the daily requirement of roughage for the *average* person.

(Although they are not yet available in the United States, they are easy enough to make at home until commercial production begins.)

One of the most common—and least popular—side effects of constipation is hemorrhoids. Nearly half of the entire nation over the age of fifty suffers from hemorrhoids—or as they are popularly known, "piles." Actually a hemorrhoid is nothing more than a big bulging vein which lies near the surface of the skin or the mucous membrane in the area of the anus.

There are two types of hemorrhoids: internal and external. The external ones are visible to the patient—with the aid of a mirror—and consist of little purplish lumps or tags around the anal opening that become swollen when the individual strains at a bowel movement. Sometimes blood clots form within the distended veins and the hemorrhoids then become tender and painful. The thin layer of skin over each hemorrhoid may even become ulcerated and bleed with every defecation.

Internal hemorrhoids, on the other hand, are rarely seen by the sufferer since they affect veins higher up in the anal canal. These veins are more extensive than the external ones and can cause considerable bleeding. Although the amount of blood lost from hemorrhoids is rarely substantial, the bleeding itself can lead to other hazards. Since cancer of the colon and rectum can *also* cause bleeding, more than one person with rectal bleeding has brushed it off as "just my hemorrhoids acting up again," neglected to see his doctor, and allowed his colon cancer to grow past the point where it could be cured.

Hemorrhoids are a major cause of pain and disability in every industrialized country on a low-roughage diet. In addition, the economic consequences from lost wages and lowered production can scarcely be calculated. The most effective treatment for hemorrhoids up until now has been surgery—relatively painful, expensive, and time-consuming. Furthermore, because hemorrhoids affect the anal area and touch the "toilet taboo" of Americans, most victims suffer in silence while spending tens of millions of dollars yearly on ointments and suppositories which *cannot possibly cure the basic problem.*

As a matter of fact, until recently, physicians were at a loss to explain exactly what caused hemorrhoids. The standard statement went something like:

"… presumably result from conditions that produce rectal venous congestion such as constipation, pregnancy, rectal disease, diarrhea, and portal hypertension."

That is hardly a definitive explanation.

As nutritional researchers around the world turned their attention to the problems of constipation, they encountered some puzzling questions. Why should constipation make the suffering of those with hemorrhoids so intense? Why should it be so out of proportion to the mechanical pressure of the hardened fecal matter pressing against the swollen veins? They then carefully retraced the route of venous drainage and made some interesting discoveries.

The purpose of the veins of the circulatory system is simply to return the blood from outlying parts of the body to the heart. The smaller veins of the anus and rectum empty into the larger veins of the pelvis just as smaller rivers drain into larger ones. On a low-roughage diet, the investigators reasoned, the dry, hardened feces that collect day after day in the colon push outward and compress the large veins nearby. This pressure acts like a dam, prevents the blood from draining out of the anal and rectal veins, and causes tremendous return pressure. The result is the swollen, inflamed, knotted veins that we call hemorrhoids.

Other investigators agreed with this finding in principle but felt there might be still another important factor causing hemorrhoids. They noted that those on low-roughage diets tend to strain and struggle to pass their small hardened stools, and in the process of straining, the pressure *within the major veins* can rise to amazing levels. For example, the pressure inside the vena cava has been measured at 300 to 400 millimeters of mercury, or about 250 to 350 percent greater than normal systolic blood pressure! This pressure is directly transmitted to the rectal and anal veins and can in itself balloon them out, weaken their walls, and result in permanent hemorrhoids.

The scientists also noted that hemorrhoids—internal or external—were rare in Africans and Asians on a traditional high-roughage diet. Obviously there is never any hard, dry fecal material to distend their colons, press on their veins, and cause the destructive return pressure. In addition, Africans and Asians never have to strain while moving their bowels. But as soon as they begin to adopt the

Western-low fiber diet, they almost invariable begin to show signs of hemorrhoids.

Clearly, there is no way to reverse the damage already done to the veins of the rectum and anus. But a high-roughage diet can help prevent bleeding, relieve the pressure within the stretched and distorted veins, and help forestall the formation of *new* hemorrhoids. It can also provide freedom from the expensive ritual of ointments, suppositories, laxatives, and all the rest of the patent medicines that hemorrhoid sufferers turn to in desperation.

Another complaint of modern life may have the same basic cause as hemorrhoids. About 10 percent of the entire population of the United States—that is, 31 million people—suffer from varicose veins. These distended veins of the legs, in addition to being annoying and unsightly, can cause swelling, muscle cramps, tension, and soreness. Occasionally they can result in open oozing and skin ulcers. But beyond that, they can even lead to potentially fatal consequences.

Let's see how the distention occurs:

Ever since man has walked on his hind legs, the body has had a difficult assignment in getting blood back to the heart from the lowest portions of the anatomy. The blood supplying the lower legs and feet is brought upward by an ingenious mechanism known as the "muscle pump." With each step the powerful muscles of the legs squeeze blood upward in the deep veins of each lower limb. But there's a catch. Each time the blood rises in the veins it tends to fall back down again. However, built into each vein is a system of valves—like locks in a canal— and every time blood is forced upward by the muscles, it is kept at that level by these valves. If these valves are somehow destroyed, the blood cannot rise effectively, it stagnates, and all the annoying and disabling symptoms of varicose veins appear.

The treatment of mild varicose veins is nonmedical—elastic stockings or support hose are generally used. But for an attractive— and still young—man or woman, elastic stockings are hardly the most appealing fashion accessory. The ultimate cure for varicose veins is still surgery—stripping out those veins with broken valves or tying off the affected veins high up on the legs.

Until recently, varicose veins have been blamed on such vague causes as standing for long periods of time. But among those people on a high-roughage diet, less than *one-tenth of one percent* suffer from varicose veins although nearly 100 percent of *them* are on their feet for long periods.

A far more likely explanation for varicose veins is the same combination of factors that cause hemorrhoids — since hemorrhoids are like varicose veins of the rectum and anus. Although a high-fiber diet may take the pressure off the large veins of the pelvis and abdomen and unblock the drainage system—thus helping the circulation of blood in the veins of the legs —there is no way that it can make the stretched and swollen veins deep within the legs go back to normal. However, restoring roughage to the diet can prevent further damage from occurring, and most important of all, it may reduce the chances of the most terrible complications of varicose veins—phlebothrombosis, thrombophlebitis, and pulmonary embolism.

Let's take the first one. "Phlebothrombosis" comes from two Greek words: *phlebo*, meaning "vein," and *thrombo*, meaning "clot." Therefore *phlebo thrombosis* means a blood clot in a vein—and that *is* a problem. As the blood begins to sludge and stagnate in the damaged deep veins of the legs, a blood clot may form. At first it is no more than a tiny blob of jellylike material poised in the blood vessel. But gradually it may acquire a "tail" stretching out behind it for some distance, and it may even become attached to the wall of the vein. Then the vein itself can become inflamed. At that point, the condition is known as "thrombophlebitis," or simply "phlebitis"— the "*-itis*" ending, as usual, indicates an inflammatory process is underway. Severe pain, swelling, and tenderness often occur at that point. But the worst is yet to come.

Without any warning the clot can suddenly break loose and race swiftly upward through progressively larger veins until it reaches the lungs, where it causes a dreaded "pulmonary embolism."

While the clot is stationary it is known as a "thrombus," but once it begins its deadly journey it becomes known as an "embolism" from the Greek word for "plug." And that's exactly what it does. That mobile clot may plug the pulmonary arteries, the vital arteries of the lungs, resulting in rapid circulatory collapse, heart failure, and death.

Unfortunately there is no way of predicting in advance when or even *if* a clot will break loose, become an embolus, and shoot upward into the lungs. That's one reason that a case of thromboembolism can be described as a "loaded shotgun aimed toward the lungs," ready to discharge dozens of blood clots into the vulnerable respiratory system.

The accepted treatment for thrombophlebitis is anticoagulants and perhaps surgically tying off the large veins toward the upper part of the leg to isolate the clots from the vital organs. However, everyone involved would agree that prevention is a far better approach. The best-known prevention—to date—consists of trying to *prevent the underlying disease.* The only known way to accomplish that is to normalize the operation of the digestive system by restoring the absent and essential roughage to the diet. That should, if the experts are right, relieve the obstruction of the large pelvic and abdominal veins and lower the pressure within the abdomen at the time of defecation, thereby preventing the stagnation of blood flow that predisposes toward clot formation.

Although nobody dies of constipation or hemorrhoids or varicose veins, they are still annoying and disabling diseases afflicting untold millions of men and women— with the small but real hazard of pulmonary embolism and its potentially fatal barrage of blood clots to the lungs.

For years these conditions were dismissed as the "penalties of civilization," but it is rapidly becoming apparent that consuming the so-called civilized diet is one of the *least* civilized things that we do. Tens of millions of Africans and Asians live their entire lives without the burdens of these diseases—and if we go back to the diet t*hat we never should have left,* so can we.

7

Two Cents A Day To Keep The Doctor Away: The Key To Survival We All Throw Away

Based on the judgments of more than 10,000 prominent medical authorities as expressed in over 20,000 medical articles and books published around the world, there is no doubt that dietary fiber or roughage is an essential part of the human diet. *To consume a "modern" low-roughage diet is to court premature death and disability.*

Lack of roughage in our diet is a deficiency—just as lack of protein or minerals is a deficiency. For a long and happy life the roughage deficiency *must* be corrected.

There are several ways of restoring adequate dietary fiber to our daily diets. First, we might switch to the staple menu of rural Africans and Asians. That means ground corn, boiled bananas, freshly dug potatoes, and plenty of beans. Most Americans would be understandably reluctant to make that kind of substitution.

The second possibility is to try and regulate our diets by selecting only those foods with the highest roughage content from the grocer's shelves. That's a very difficult assignment—for a couple of reasons. Nearly 90 percent of the most common 50,000 items stocked by the average supermarket have had nearly every scrap of roughage removed in the refining or manufacturing process. Here are some examples:

1. "Instant" potatoes, "instant" rice, cake mixes, puddings, desserts, gravies, stuffings, cereals, and the like have been stripped of dietary fiber.
2. Bread, pastry, commercial baked goods, and "convenience" items containing ultra-refined flour are nearly all uniformly low in dietary fiber.

To convert the average American diet to a high-roughage diet would require the following changes:

1. Use only whole-grain products such as whole wheat, rolled oats, and brown rice.
2. Consume *fresh* fruits and vegetables raw or barely cooked with seeds, strings, and skins intact, if at all possible.
3. Cut to a bare minimum consumption of refined sugar, soft drinks, fats, and meat.

The vast majority of American families will reject that regimen since they have been conditioned to the "fashionable" and seductive low-roughage routine. Beyond that, there is an important element of reality. With food prices already sky-high, few individuals or families can afford the approximately 30 percent additional cost of converting their daily fare to the ideal high-roughage diet. But that doesn't mean they have to suffer the agonies of heart attacks or colon cancer or all the rest of the roughage-deficiency diseases. There is an easy and appetizing way out.

Look at it this way. Our goal is to fortify the average American diet by bringing the roughage level up to about twenty-four grams each day. Since our diet contains approximately six grams of dietary fiber already, there is a daily deficit of about eighteen grams of roughage, or just a little over half an ounce. What we need is a palatable, wholesome, and inexpensive source of dietary fiber. We need something that can be added to our daily diet almost as easily as a vitamin pill to bring our roughage consumption right up to normal. Many such products have been tested, and the one that seems to fit the requirement best of all is a natural part of each grain of wheat that is usually discarded in the milling process or used as animal fodder. It is called "bran," and it makes up the first six layers of outer coating of the wheat berry.

Wheat bran is inexpensive and a pound is about a month's supply. As a source of roughage, bran is outstanding—it is 12 percent dietary fiber and is five times as effective in restoring roughage to the body as whole-wheat flour. That means a small amount added to the daily diet pays handsome dividends in protection.

It's easy to determine the correct amount of bran necessary to restore the roughage to the diet of each person. The simplest way is to start with a small amount each day and gradually increase it until the desired results are obtained.

For the average adult that might mean about two teaspoons three times a day. Some individuals require as much as three *tablespoons* daily while others do well on one *teaspoon* three times a day. Children between five and thirteen should be started on half the minimum ration, that is, half a teaspoon three times a day. Children between three and five need about half a teaspoon *daily* on the average.

There is an almost infallible way to tell when the ideal amount of bran is being consumed. When the bowel movement is large in amount, well-formed, low in odor, and passed without straining once (or twice) a day, the roughage in the diet is just right. For the first week or so there may be an increase in the amount of gas passed and there may also be a feeling of fullness after consuming the bran. Those are two important signs that the extra fiber is doing its job. If there is any difficulty passing the bowel movement, the amount of bran should be *gradually* increased, say at the rate of an extra teaspoon a day. If the movements become loose or too frequent, it's a sign to cut down on the bran.

The next question is: "What's the best way to take the bran?" That requires some explanation. The most desirable form of bran comes in the form of dry flakes that are easily adapted to anyone's daily diet. Some people prefer to take their bran dry, washing it down with a glass of water or fruit juice. There are, however, dozens of easy and attractive ways to get your daily roughage requirement. For example, you can:

1. Sprinkle it over a dry breakfast cereal with milk.

2. Mix it with cooked cereal, before or after cooking.

3. Add it to your orange juice or other fruit juice.

4. Mix it with yogurt—any flavor.

5. Add it to soups.

6. Mix it with applesauce.

7. Combine it with ground meat to make hamburgers, meat loaf, stuffed peppers, etc.

8. Add it to any home-baked bread or pastry.

9. Include it (as I have done) in any of the sample recipes in **Chapter 10**.

Within the first seven days you will begin to enjoy the benefits of having restored the essential roughage to your diet. Constipation should vanish promptly. Those who suffered from hemorrhoids or other anal/rectal problems may find relief. Victims of diverticulosis—*after obtaining their doctor's consent to adding roughage*—should feel an almost immediate improvement. (You may want to ask your doctor to read "Unprocessed Bran in Treatment of Diverticular Disease of the Colon" in the *British Medical Journal* [1972j, Vol. 2, pp. 137-140.) Those with elevated cholesterol levels may want to have their blood cholesterol checked just *before* they use bran to correct their roughage deficiency and then have their doctor repeat the test in six weeks: The results should be gratifying and reassuring for both doctor and patient. (Once again, a good source for your doctor might be "Utilization of Wheat by Adult Man," *American Journal of Clinical Nutrition* 24: 181-193.)

Although, as we have seen, no diet in the world is going to reverse the physical changes that are evident in varicose veins, when a person no longer has to strain with each bowel movement, the tremendous pressure that such straining generates is absent and the damaged veins can function much better. At the same time, further vein damage is prevented. ***Anyone suffering from a severe disease such as kidney disease, diabetes, etc., must have absolute permission from his or her physician before consuming bran.***

Another bonus comes in the battle against obesity (see **Chapter 8**). Bran can be included in nearly every weight-reduction diet—with your doctor's approval, as usual. Being able to eat something three times a day that is chewable, has body, and provides a feeling of fullness —without significant calories—is a dieter's dream come true.

The last benefit of returning to a high-roughage diet is difficult to explain. It's a kind of indescribable feeling of well-being, the realization that finally, after many years, your body is functioning the way it was designed to function. People who have followed the diet characterize that sensation as "feeling like a machine that's humming along," or "alert and energetic the way I was twenty years ago," or simply, "alive again." When you experience the sensation, you'll understand.

An important question is: "How long should I stay on the high-roughage diet?" The best answer is: "Only as long as you want to feel good." As you notice your appetite for semisynthetic junk food beginning to wane and your appreciation of wholesome food begin to increase, the high-fiber diet will become a way of life. Actually this question answers itself, because after a month on a normal high-fiber diet, there will be no way that you can be convinced to go back to the unappealing low-roughage way of life. Try it and you'll see.

Now let's get down to the specifics of *how* to restore the roughage to our diet. Since not everyone has the same life style, there are three separate high-roughage diet plans.

The first one is the "ideal," but since we don't live in an "ideal world," the other two are only slightly less effective:

High-Roughage Diet Plan Number One: "The Ideal"

AVOID: Refined sugar and refined sugar products including sweets, candy, and ice cream as much as possible.

SUBSTITUTE: Unprocessed honey, unprocessed molasses, sugar-containing fruit (dates, apples, pears, bananas, etc.) Fruit juices instead of soft drinks, home-baked whole-grain pastry made with honey.

NOTE: The reason for avoiding refined sugar is that there is some important evidence that refined sugar alters the dominant type of bacteria present in the colon and increases the possibility of colon and rectal cancer. It also may contribute to the elevation of blood cholesterol.

AVOID: All refined flour products.

SUBSTITUTE: Whole-grain-flour products such as whole-wheat bread, whole-wheat crackers, whole-wheat pastries, pies and cakes.

NOTE: Whole-wheat pastry flour is available for home bakers. That makes it possible to prepare everything from cookies to pie crusts with whole-grain flour. Commercial bakery goods made from whole-grain products exist, but are expensive, and may be hard to find.

AVOID: All refined cereal products which are sugar or honey-coated and pre-sweetened. Rice-based cereals are especially low in fiber, including puffed rice, and the others like them. "Instant" and "quick-cooking" products also may be deficient in roughage. That may include instant grits, instant oatmeal, instant rice, instant breading, instant stuffing, and a high proportion of the over one hundred and fifty boxed breakfast cereals.

SUBSTITUTE: Whole-grain cereal products such as whole wheat, brown rice, whole-grain corn meal (masa), 100 percent rye flour, and carob flour.

Some of the boxed cereals, although they tend to be expensive, are relatively high in fiber:

1. 100 percent bran cereal
2. Bran flakes (40 percent bran)
3. Bran flakes with raisins
4. Most granola cereals
5. Wheat flakes
6. Puffed wheat
7. Shredded wheat
8. Dry oat cereals without added sweetener

The outstanding disadvantage of some boxed cereals—including some of the intensively advertised so-called natural products—is that they may contain up to 25 percent (or more) refined sugar. (Even brown sugar is *refined* sugar.) That tends to undercut their value as a source of fiber.

AVOID: All overprocessed fruits and vegetables, including canned, frozen, and other "prepared" versions. (Dried fruit is an exception: it is high in fiber.)

SUBSTITUTE: Fresh fruits and vegetables eaten with as little peeling, cooking, and processing as possible.

NOTE: As a source of roughage, vegetables are *not* as effective as whole cereal grains. However, they have an important place in the "ideal" high-roughage diet.

AVOID: "Convenience" snack foods made with white flour. They may include various pizza-flavored, onion-flavored and cheese-flavored cracker-type chips, crisps, and twists.

SUBSTITUTE: Tortilla chips if made from whole corn and water, *any kind of nuts*, popcorn, whole-grain pretzels, sunflower seeds, pumpkin seeds, dried fruit, toasted soybeans, toasted wheat, raisins.

NOTE: A lot of natural snacks are perfectly suited to a high-roughage diet. If you think about it for a moment, it makes sense. Most traditional snack foods are primitive seeds or grains which humans have been consuming for 50,000 years or more. Perhaps there is something in the wisdom of the body that constantly drives us back to these high-roughage basic nuts, seeds, and grains.

Special situations: "Ethnic" dishes are an oasis of high roughage foods in a desert of low-roughage commodities. They have survived the passage of time virtually unchanged and offer an excellent way of adding roughage to the diet in an interesting and appetizing way. A few examples follow:

Middle East: *Bulgur* is high-roughage cracked wheat.

Russian: *Kasha* is buckwheat groats, high in fiber.

Mexican: Authentic *tortillas* are made from high-roughage whole corn ground with lime water. The shells of *tacos, enchiladas,* and *tostadas,* if made faithfully, are of the same ingredients.

Italian: Whole-wheat *pasta* is easily available in Italy; with some searching it can be found elsewhere. Homemade *pizza* can be prepared with whole-wheat flour.

German: Breading, stuffing, dumplings, and gravy can all be prepared with whole-wheat flour.

Sunday morning favorites like waffles, pancakes, and French toast can make an excellent contribution to the daily roughage quota if they are prepared with wholegrain products.

Baby food is a very special consideration. Generally processed beyond recognition and thickened with generous amounts of low-roughage tapioca flour, many are aimed at Mommy's taste buds. However, there is an oasis of *relatively* high fiber in the panoply of commercial baby food. A list of those highest in roughage follows:

BABY CEREAL

1. Barley
2. High protein
3. Mixed cereal
4. Oatmeal cereal

BABY DINNERS (in jars or cans)

1. Beef noodle dinner
2. Macaroni, tomatoes, meat, and cereal dinner
3. Split peas, vegetables, ham or bacon dinner
4. Vegetables and bacon with cereal dinner
5. Vegetables and beef with cereal dinner
6. Vegetables and chicken with cereal dinner
7. Vegetables and ham with cereal dinner

FRUITS AND VEGETABLES (in jars or cans)

1. Pears
2. Green beans
3. Strained peas
4. Squash

However, as soon as the doctor suggests that the baby is ready for baby food, ask him to approve "real" fruit and vegetables prepared in the family blender. But be sure to get your doctor's approval before adding or subtracting anything from the diet of an infant.

As you can see, Diet Plan Number One requires total commitment to the idea of a natural high-roughage diet. Even with all the fiber it contains, it will probably still be necessary to add about one teaspoon of unprocessed bran to the diet, one to three times a day, to reach the goal of well-formed, low-odor bowel movements passed without straining. (Incidentally, the *relative* lack of odor to the feces results from several factors. On the high-roughage diet there is less decomposition of bile acids, the bacteria in the colon are different, and smaller amounts of refined sugar cut down on putrefaction of the contents of the colon.)

For those who are unable to make the necessary sacrifices—both in time and money—to follow the "ideal" diet plan, there is a reasonable compromise:

High-Roughage Diet Plan Number Two

Basically this consists of following Diet Plan Number One for *seven days*, then switching to Diet Plan Number Three. This approach helps the digestive system to make a rapid transition from the stagnant low-roughage operation to the fast-processing and prompt elimination of a high-roughage diet.

Realistically speaking, there are still many people who will be unable to follow the *ideal* diet even for a week. Because of the cost or the necessity to totally revamp their system of food preparation, they need another way to conquer their roughage deficiency. The best solution for them is:

High-Roughage Diet Plan Number Three

This involves starting right off—today if possible—by supplementing the diet with unprocessed bran in sufficient amounts to insure normal digestion and adequate protection from heart attacks, cancer of the colon and rectum, and the other conditions that result from a low-roughage diet.

Certainly you can improve the efficiency of your diet if you add fresh fruit and vegetables, whole-grain products, and eliminate most of the refined sugar. However, even *if you continue to eat a low-roughage overprocessed typical American diet*, you will obtain most of the benefits and *most* of the protection of a high-roughage diet by simply taking your bran three times a day. That makes it ideal for students, working wives, traveling salesmen, men and women in the military, and everyone else who just can't control their daily menu as much as they would like.

In **Chapters 9** and **10**, there are many sample diets and recipes and useful hints that allow bran to be "smuggled" unnoticed, into the diets of even the most fastidious eaters. Whichever diet plan you choose, from the simplest to the most elaborate, you can be sure that you will eat better, feel better, look better, and based on the findings of tens of thousands of medical experts around the world you can look forward to a longer, happier, and healthier life.

8

Obesity: An Avoidable Illness

During the past hundred years a strange and terrible epidemic of a life-threatening disease has spread over our nation. The name of that disease is *obesity*, and it threatens to shorten the lives of nearly *two hundred million Americans*. Of all the threats to our national health, obesity is probably the most neglected and least understood—and potentially among the most lethal.

According to insurance company calculations, a person over the age of forty-five who carries as little as *ten extra pounds* decreases his chances of survival by about 8 percent. For every additional pound of excess weight, his risk of dying prematurely rises approximately *1 percent*. The individual who is twenty pounds overweight has a 20 percent greater chance of perishing prematurely, and a man carrying fifty additional pounds has a *56 percent* greater likelihood of an early demise.

Obesity tips the scales of survival against its victims in two ways:

1. Excessive weight makes a person more vulnerable to potentially fatal diseases such as diabetes, heart attacks, high blood pressure and thromboembolism (blood clots that can travel to the lungs with deadly effects).
2. Overweight produces a significantly higher death rate from such conditions as diabetes, inflammation of the kidneys, cirrhosis of the liver, gall bladder conditions, appendicitis, and

postoperative complications. In addition, obese people are more likely to develop varicose veins, arthritis, and the various complications of pregnancy. (It is *not* a coincidence that appendicitis, varicose veins, thromboembolism, phlebitis, and heart attacks have all been associated with our national roughage-deficient diet.)

The worst part about it is that most Americans *hate* to be overweight. They know instinctively that extra fat is unhealthy and unappealing. And they spend billions each year in a desperate battle against extra pounds. They buy costly "dietetic" foods, pay dues at health clubs and reducing salons, and most expensive of all, seek medical help in losing weight.

The only problem is that until recently there was very little a doctor could offer a patient who was serious about reducing. The standard approach was usually a pat on the back and the kindly suggestion to "cut down," get more exercise, and avoid sweets. Alternately, the overweight person could visit high-pressure weight-reduction clinics that guaranteed to take off a certain number of pounds for a stiff fee. Both techniques have one thing in common— they rarely produce any *long-term benefit*. Almost anyone can lose weight on almost any kind of diet— but keeping the weight off is where virtually every popular diet program fails. The all-too-familiar story is:

Adhere to a rigid diet, lose weight, go back to eating "normally," and watch the pounds *relentlessly return*. Over 90 percent of those who lose weight—whether by diet or drugs—gain back every pound, and often more for good measure.

The great irony of our time is that while Americans are begrudging themselves ten calories here and twenty calories there and desperately struggling to limit their carbohydrates to thirty grams a day, millions of others around the world are consuming up to *three thousand calories* daily and *six hundred grams of carbohydrate* without gaining an ounce! Rural Africans and Asians, for example, remain lean and lithe throughout their lifetimes on high-calorie, high-carbohydrate diets.

Understanding their secret promises to free more than a hundred million citizens from the bondage of obesity and the ever-present threat of the diseases that obesity brings on. As medical researchers pursued their study of the role of roughage in the diet, they made the following observations:

1. Virtually all those in our society who are obese got that way on a *low-roughage* diet featuring refined sugar and ultra-refined white flour products.
2. Many patients complain that although they adhere to the prescribed low-calorie diets, they fail to lose weight, and even continue to gain. (Alibis aside, every experienced physician has observed this.)
3. Throughout the world there are individuals and groups who consume high-calorie diets *without* developing obesity. They include strict vegetarians and rural Asians and Africans.
4. As recently as two hundred years ago in Europe, obesity was rare.

After careful study and analysis of tens of thousands of individual diets, scientists developed the following explanations:

1. Because it is so seductively appetizing (high in refined sugar and ultra-processed flour), the low-roughage diet literally compels overconsumption, making obesity almost *inevitable*. Ice cream, cake mixes, commercial baked goods, canned fruits, soda pop, and commercial desert products are low in bulk, high in sweetness, and can be eaten in massive quantities. Energetic advertising of these high-profit items also encourages excessive consumption—especially by the least discerning and most vulnerable members of our society, our children.
2. The typical "treatment" of obesity is to place the patient on a *low-calorie* diet. That diet is almost invariably also a *low-roughage* diet. Here are three typical meals on a medically approved reducing diet:

BREAKFAST

½ cup orange juice

1 boiled egg
1 slice toast (from ultra-refined flour)
Tea or coffee

LUNCH

1 frankfurter
1 roll (from ultra-refined flour)
Celery and radishes
Tea or coffee

DINNER

3 ounces of roast beef
1 cup spinach
½ cup carrots
Tea or coffee

That adds up to a grand total of approximately 720 calories, or just about one-third of what the average person needs just to maintain his weight; theoretically it should produce as much as a three-pound-a-week weight loss, week after week. Yet after a token initial loss, many patients are unable to lose weight on this calorie-deficient diet.

The explanation that has evaded doctors for so long may actually be obvious: This type of reducing diet is distressingly deficient in dietary fiber. As confirmation, nearly all patients who suffer on this and similar diets are notably *constipated*. That in itself should have been a clue that the normal operation of the digestive system was being impaired rather than helped.

3. Obesity is rare in *strict* vegetarians, those who consume only fruits, nuts, vegetables, and the like, and who forsake even eggs and milk. Rural Africans and Asians may eat as much as 3,000 calories daily, but since their diets, like the vegetarians' diets, are *high in roughage*, they almost never become overweight.

4. In Europe, before 1770, a low-roughage diet was expensive and difficult to obtain—only the wealthy could *afford* to get fat. The poor consumed mostly flour and cereal products—high in *calories* and high in *roughage*—*and* remained thin.

One of the most-promoted diets in recent history is the so-called low-carbohydrate diet. Untold millions of Americans have tried it in one form or another—with varying results. Although it has been around for many years under many names, the low-carbohydrate diet has always attracted converts because it promises, "You will never be hungry!"

But the basic problem with the low-carbohydrate diet is that it does half the right thing for the wrong reason. Based on the observation that the American diet is high in carbohydrates, this popular diet attempts to eliminate most (if not all) carbohydrates from the daily menu. They begin with a goal of "zero" carbohydrates—an impossibility—and then move on to a ration of about one ounce or thirty grams of carbohydrates daily. The promoters of the various diets correctly point out that the average ineffective reducing diet may contain as much as three hundred grams of carbohydrates a day—or more. So, they reason, remove the carbohydrates, and the weight must come down.

But they are at a loss to explain why Africans can consume as much as 3,000 calories a day, including *six hundred grams of carbohydrates*, without ever becoming obese. Carbohydrates are obviously not the basic problem—*lack of roughage is*. Once these same Africans adopt our notorious low-fiber diet, they put on weight as much as we do. The story is told of the British medical missionary who recently returned to Africa after being away for many years. When his plane landed at the airport near his former mission, he was amazed and appalled to see, for the first time in his life, groups of *fat* Africans.

He investigated further and confirmed that the only basic changes that had occurred in their diet during the past forty years were the addition of refined sugar and ultra- processed white flour. As a matter of fact, the *first* authenticated heart attack in all of East Africa did not occur until *1956*—*in* an African who had adopted a Western diet.

It's only in the past four or five years that medical experts have begun to gain some real understanding of why people become fat. Detailed and sophisticated observations of obese individuals indicate that they have entirely different eating habits from those who have no trouble maintaining their normal weight. Those who tend to become overweight often have a delayed "satisfaction response." That is, they can consume massive quantities of food before they get the signal from their appetite control center that they aren't hungry any more. Normal eaters, on the other hand, reach the stage of "fullness" much more rapidly—and quickly curtail their intake.

Those who tend to be obese generally consume their food quickly, chew it superficially, and have a taste for items which pack a lot of calories into a small package. In addition, their digestive system seems to operate at peak efficiency, extracting every last calorie from their daily menu. For those people, a high-roughage diet seems ideal. *In effect it counteracts each and every one of these obesity-enhancing mechanisms.* Let's take a look:

1. A high-roughage diet is harder to eat. Instant mashed potatoes and cottony white bread slide down like so much slush. But brown rice, raw carrots, sliced cucumbers, and fresh apples require time and energy to chew and absorb. A person on a high-fiber diet is much more likely to reach the point of satisfaction before he eats too much.

2. A high-roughage diet is much bulkier than a low-roughage diet. By the time an individual does away with a big plate of lettuce or half a bunch of celery, plus a serving of meat loaf laced with bran and a side order of peas, he is hardly in the mood for a heaping bowl of white-flour spaghetti and a couple of slices of white bread.

3. As the items in a high-roughage diet are chewed, large amounts of saliva and gastric juices are produced. This additional liquid mixes with the food in the stomach and causes swelling of the fibers in the food. That distends the stomach and gives prompt and lasting feeling of "fullness"— that often evasive feeling that so many dieters say they miss.

4. There is some convincing—although not yet conclusive— evidence that a diet with abundant roughage actually impairs the ability of the small intestine to *absorb* calories. That might mean that someone on a high-roughage diet can actually *eat more and still lose.*

5. It has been well established that those who consume a high-fiber diet actually excrete more fat in each bowel movement

than those on the low- roughage diet. A dieter on a high-roughage diet can rejoice in the knowledge that he is excreting a portion of his excess body fat as each day on his diet goes by.

6. The bran portion of the high-fiber diet is a dieter's dream come true. It provides something which he can *eat* and chew three times a day without risking even an ounce of extra weight.

7. Finally, a high-roughage reducing diet eliminates the bane of nearly every weight reduction program—constipation. *No one on a high-fiber diet is going to be constipated.*

A high-roughage weight-reduction diet benefits the dieter in two other ways. It takes off weight, thus reducing the hazard of developing diseases like heart attack, thromboembolism, and all the rest. At the same time, it acts directly on the body to blockade the specific mechanisms that produce these (and other) serious conditions. Most important of all, the high-roughage weight-reduction diet is a diet of abundance, not deficiency. Instead of starving your body into abnormally disposing of the accumulated fat, you eat yourself into a condition of normal weight distribution. At the same time, you can bypass drugs, shots, pills, and all the risks that go along with them.

All you need to do is follow the High-Roughage Reducing Diet that follows this chapter. Provided you eat nothing but the items listed and you avoid all refined sugar and our-processed flour products, you should slowly and *effortlessly* begin to lose weight. The excess fat will come off gradually—and that's an advantage, for two reasons. First, losing large amounts of body weight too quickly can be dangerous to your health. Secondly, the ideal high-roughage reducing diet is a diet without hunger and without *any deprivation whatsoever.* You can stay on it as long as you want to— preferably for life. Your weight will slowly come down to the ideal level and—as long as you adhere to the diet— stay there. Does it really work? The answer to that is that the diet has been thoroughly tested by many billions of people over the past fifty thousand years. *It is the normal, natural, rational diet of mankind.*

Obesity is a terrible disease—but it is a relatively new disease as far as the history of the human race is concerned. To overcome it, all we have to do is *restore our diets to what they were before obesity existed.*

9

The High-Roughage Reducing Diet

The basic principle of this reducing diet is to normalize the functioning of the digestive system—not to derange it as most other weight-reduction diets do. To ensure your success, there are some important principles to follow:

1. Be certain that your doctor agrees that you are in good health; a recent physical exam is essential.
2. Those who are already suffering from nutritionally-oriented diseases such as, diabetes, high blood pressure, heart disease, diverticular disease, kidney disease, and others should not undertake *any* diet without their doctor's specific permission and approval.
3. The High-Roughage Reducing Diet must be followed exactly and precisely. There are no exceptions, no "days off," and no corners to cut. Warning: Addition of excessive fat or ultra-processed starches or refined sugars will result in failure of the diet.
4. The basic principle of the diet is simply to overcome the fiber deficiency in the so-called "modern" diet and make normal digestion possible *for the first time in your life*. Once your body is given the chance to operate the way it was designed to, it will automatically regulate itself within the normal range.

When you begin to eat adequate roughage, the following dramatic changes should take place:

1. The bacteria in your colon will shift to the lactobacillus-streptococcus forms which encourage *normal* fermentation of the food which you consume, rather than the abnormal fermentation of the low-roughage diet.
2. The amount of fat and fatty acid which you excrete in your bowel movement should increase significantly.
3. The rate of absorption of the food that you consume should decline.
4. The level of lipids ("fat") in your blood should diminish.

There are five very important things to remember to assure the success of this diet program:

1. *Eat slowly.* The fiber which you consume must have time to absorb the liquid in your diet to provide that essential feeling of fullness and satisfaction.
2. *Don't eat unless you are hungry.* Many obese/overweight people interpret the typical eat-all-you-want diet as a challenge—and one which they rise to meet. Only eat as much as you need to feel satisfied.
3. *Drink plenty of water.* Fiber needs water in order to make your body work the way it should. Since you lose about four glasses a day in perspiration, urine, and feces, you need at least eight glasses a day for dieting purposes—and a little more won't hurt.
4. *Don't cheat.* If you really want to lose weight, this diet can help you, but it won't do a thing for you unless you stay on it. Sabotaging the diet only sabotages you, your appearance, and your health.
5. *Remember that this is not a "diet" in the usual sense.* You are only getting around to eating—finally—the way you should have been eating all these years. **Billions** of others around the world have lived their entire lives on this kind of diet without suffering any of the illnesses and disabilities that you have come to take for granted. If they can do it, so can you.

The menu plan of the High-Roughage Reducing Diet is simple and straightforward:

1. Eliminate all low-roughage foods, all ultra-processed flour products, and all refined sugar.
2. Eat high-roughage foods, including whole-grain cereal products, high-fiber fruits and vegetables, and nuts and seeds whenever possible.
3. Eat moderate amounts of low-fat meat, fish, and poultry. (Incidentally, as you restore the roughage to your diet, you will be amazed to find that you no longer crave large amounts of meat.)
4. Use moderate amounts of fats and oils for cooking and salads.
5. Substitute molasses and honey for refined sugar.
6. Reduce "hot" spices and relishes to the minimum. There are two reasons for this. First, "hot" spices tend to increase consumption of cereal grain products—from brown rice to hamburger rolls. Second, most relishes such as ketchup, steak sauces, pickle relish, etc., are high in refined sugar.
7. All flour products should be made from one of the following types of flour exclusively:
   - whole-grain rye flour
   - whole-wheat flour
   - soy flour
   - whole ground corn meal
   - buckwheat flour (whole grain)

   Bread should contain only these flours without added refined sugar and a minimum of shortening. Other flour products should be made in a similar way. (See the recipes in **Chapter 10**.) Many of these items can be purchased ready-made in health-food stores—but read the labels carefully to be sure that they contain only these flours and no added refined sugar. (One of the ironies of "modern" merchandising is that we can purchase our daily diet in two kinds of stores: "health-food" stores and—by implication—"unhealthy" food stores.)
8. Avoid all "synthetic" products; they are invariably low roughage and will interfere with your diet success. That

includes items like non-dairy creamer, synthetic whipped topping, artificial sour cream, and imitation *anything*.

9. Do not eat any of the high-sugar, high-starch items that clutter menus everywhere. They include all "commercial" baked goods, ice cream, ice milk, imitation ice cream, imitation ice milk, sherbet, "commercial" candy, sugar-containing soft drinks, pre-sweetened cereals, and all other products containing ultra-processed flour, and/or refined sugar.

10. Unfortunately, there is no place for alcoholic beverages on this diet—or on any other medically-sound diet, for that matter. Ethyl alcohol, the kind that is in all "alcoholic" beverages, is swiftly converted to sugar in the body. It is low-roughage (an understatement) and will undermine the entire diet plan. There is, however, one consolation. Many of those who have followed the high-roughage diet plan find that within a week to a month their desire for alcohol has almost totally disappeared. In any event, there is no way around it—high roughage is "The Thinking Man's Diet," not "The Drinking Man's Diet."

11. Fruits and vegetables should be eaten raw if possible—otherwise, with the absolute minimum amount of cooking and with seeds, skins, and strings as intact as you can manage.

12. An indispensable part of the diet is the addition of unprocessed bran in the average amount of two teaspoonfuls three times a day.

A sample menu looks something like this:

BREAKFAST

(2 teaspoons bran with a full glass of water before eating)

Fruit: Raw apple or pear (eaten with the skin) or an orange
Cereal: 1 serving all-bran or shredded wheat or puffed oats plus a small amount of milk and honey
1 egg

Whole-wheat toast (100 percent stone-ground whole wheat)

Tea or coffee (Use honey instead of sugar and a small amount of milk if desired.)

LUNCH

(2 teaspoons bran with a full glass of water before eating)

Roast-beef sandwich consisting of two small slices roast beef on whole-wheat bread (100 percent stone ground)
Lettuce and tomato on the above sandwich, if desired
Carrot sticks and sliced green pepper
Strawberries for dessert (no sugar or cream—small amount of honey if desired) Use *fresh* strawberries only.
Tea or coffee (Use honey instead of sugar and a small amount of milk if desired.)

DINNER

(2 teaspoons bran with a full glass of water before eating)

Homemade pea soup
Broiled chicken (Fat under the skin may be removed.)
Brown rice
Corn on the cob
Blueberries for dessert (No sugar or cream—use a small amount of milk if desired.) Use fresh blueberries only. (Only fresh fruits should be used since the canned and frozen varieties *usually* contain additional sugar.)

BEDTIME SNACK 1

Cup freshly-popped popcorn (not microwave)—no butter or oil, a small amount of salt

You will notice some interesting things about this diet. Generally, no amounts are specified. There are two reasons for that. First, anyone who *really* wants to lose weight will eat as little as necessary to feel "full" so that they can reach their goal. Secondly, within sensible limits, as long as the diet is high in roughage, one cup or two cups of all-bran cereal or an extra helping of meat or brown rice is not going to make that much difference over the long run. Let me emphasize again that this is not a lose-twenty pounds-then-eat-yourself-crazy diet program. *This is a lifetime menu plan designed to restore your body to its normal functioning and incidentally to its normal weight.*

An important addition to the diet is two tablespoons of live-bacteria yogurt daily to help convert the intestinal bacteria to the lactobacillus forms which do not tend to split the bile acids nor cause other potentially serious problems. *But* the brand of yogurt must have live bacterial cultures…otherwise it won't do its job. (Read the label carefully.)

You can make up your own menu from the following groups of foods. In the process keep these things in mind:

1. The success of your weight-reduction program depends on you. If you cheat, you are cheating yourself.

2. Keep the amounts moderate—sufficient to be fully satisfying but no more than that.

3. Be vigilant to keep refined sugars, low-roughage flours and cereal products, and large amounts of fats from creeping into the diet.

4. Be patient. On this diet you can avoid hunger and the rest of "dieting discomfort"—you don't have to rush. Remember, a weight loss of only half a pound a week adds up to *twenty-six* pounds a year.

Use the following food lists to make up your personal diet plan.

I. MILK PRODUCTS—use in moderation. Whole milk , Cheese, Skim Milk, Yogurt

II. VEGETABLES—any vegetable on this list, in moderation. Prepare any way except fried. Do not add oil or butter except in very small amounts. Cook as little as possible and consume seed, skins, and strings if possible.

Artichoke, Beans— white, pinto, brown, green, wax, red, black, lima, yellow ...

Beets, Beet greens, Broccoli, Brussels Sprouts, Cabbage, Carrots, Cauliflower, Chestnuts, Garbanzos, Collard greens, Corn on the cob, Black-eyed peas, Eggplant, Kale, Kohlrabi, Lentils, Lamb's-Quarters, Mustard greens, Okra, Onions, Parsley, Parsnips, Peas, Green Peppers, Rutabagas, Sweet Potatoes, Turnips, Salsify, Kelp, Spinach, Winter Squash, Potatoes, Turnip Greens, Frozen Mixed Vegetables, Yams.

III. FRUIT—to be eaten raw, with skin *if possible*.

Raw Apples, Berries, Dried Litchis, Dried Apples Blackberries, Longans, Dried Apricots, Blueberries, Loquats, Avocados, Boysenberries, Olives, Cherimoya, Cranberries, Dried peaches, Citrus Fruits, Elderberries, Pears, Coconut, Gooseberries, Dried Pears, Currants, Loganberries, Prunes, Figs, Raspberries, Persimmons, Guavas, Strawberries, Raisins.

IV. ANIMAL PROTEIN—Cook any way *except* fried. Eat moderate amounts.

Beef—carefully trimmed of all visible fat.

Veal—carefully trimmed of all visible fat.

Organ meats of any species—liver, heart, kidneys, brains, sweetbreads, tripe, tongue. Remove all visible fat.

Pork—lean and carefully trimmed of all visible fat.

Chicken, duck, turkey—remove all fat from under skin *before* cooking.

Fish

Eggs

V. CEREAL, GRAINS AND SEEDS

Bran cereals (without added sweetener)

Buckwheat

Bulgur

Puffed-Oat cereal (without added sweetener)

Brown Rice

Whole Sesame Seeds

Hot breakfast cereals made from wheat (except "quick-cooking" and "instant" forms)

Dried breakfast cereals made from wheat (except those coated with sugar and/or honey)

Shredded Wheat (without added sweetener)

Wild Rice

VI. BREAD AND FLOURS
Pumpernickel bread (100 percent rye pumpernickel only)
Whole-wheat bread (100 percent stone ground only)
Corn bread (made from whole-grain ground corn meal)
Rye bread (100 percent rye only)
Tortillas (from whole ground corn only)
100 percent rye flour
Soy flour
Buckwheat flour (whole grain)
100 percent stone-ground whole-wheat flour
Whole-grain ground corn flour
Carob flour

VII. NUTS—These should be purchased without added sugar, salt, or oil. They are usually labeled "raw" although they may have been roasted, not fried.

Peanuts, Pecans, Pignolia Nuts, Pistachios, Popcorn, Sunflower Seeds, Walnuts, Almonds, Beechnuts, Brazil Nuts, Cashews, Hazelnuts

VIII. CAFFEINE-CONTAINING BEVERAGES
Powdered Breakfast Cocoa (*not* cocoa mix with sugar added)
Tea (Use only honey as a sweetener.)
These seven food lists can be combined in the following ways:

BREAKFAST

(one item from each list indicated) PLUS 2 teaspoons of bran with a full glass of water before eating.

List III-one item
List IV-one item
List V-one item
List VI-one item
Coffee or Tea or Cocoa

LUNCH

(one item from each list) 2 teaspoons of bran List II - one item

List III - one item
List IV - one item
List V - one item
List VI - one item
Coffee or Tea or Cocoa

DINNER

(one item from each list, except two from List II) 2 teaspoons of bran with a full glass of water before eating

List I - one item
List II - two items
List III - one item (for dessert)
List IV - one item
List VII - one item–snack at bedtime
Coffee or Tea or Cocoa

Remember, eat only *moderate* amounts.

NOTE: Unrefined sweeteners include molasses, honey, and cleaned "raw" sugar.("Brown" sugar is *refined* sugar. It should not be used.)

There is another benefit of the High Roughage Diet that deserves comment. Nearly all overeating is motivated at least in part by emotional factors. Tension, anxiety, the excessively fast pace of our daily lives—all encourage overeating. There seems to be something about a high-roughage diet which induces an internal feeling of calmness and tranquility. After a week or so on the program, that compulsion to rush and to argue and to worry seems to diminish. Most people find it easier to fall asleep at night and they feel more refreshed upon awakening. The tranquilizing effect of the high-roughage diet is only based on individual reports and has not yet been scientifically validated. Make your own observations from your own experience.

Whenever you decide to lose weight, the High-Roughage Diet is there to help you. But you should be aware of one thing—it is *habit-forming*. After suffering the deprivation and disappointment of previous weight-reduction programs, the pleasure of feeling satisfied, knowing your body is finally functioning as it should—and losing weight in the process—may make it impossible to ever go back to your old low-roughage ways of eating.

10

High-Roughage Recipes And Menu Hints

Although bran may appear a little formidable at first—it looks so brown and dry—it really can be a cook's best friend. Each bran flake soaks up moisture like a tiny sponge and if you just give the liquid time to soak in—two or three minutes is fine—the "roughage" becomes "softage" and makes the dish moist and full-bodied.

Cooking with bran has another important advantage—especially these days—since it is an ideal thickener and extender. It's much cheaper than commercial bread crumbs, and it has much more body than flour so it makes meat dishes and canned foods go that much farther.

This section is divided into two parts. First of all, there's the "quick and easy" section. Sometimes there just isn't enough time to clear off the counter-space and cook a meal from scratch—especially if you have small children. So I've worked out some ideas that will let you change food right off the supermarket shelf into "instant" high roughage. Of course, that's not the ideal way to do it, but getting your roughage that way is certainly better than not getting it at all. Just be sure to mix well and wait a minute or so to let the bran soak up the liquid, and you won't even know it's there!

Canned Goods - You can add about a tablespoon of bran per serving with no trouble at all. That supplies half the daily roughage allowance for each person. It also gives the dish a fuller flavor and makes it more satisfying at the same time. Incidentally, don't put too much faith in the number of servings specified on the can label—those canners always seem to come from families of light eaters. Just use your own judgment.

Canned Soups -Fairly thick soups like cream of mushroom, cream of celery, cream of turkey, pea soup, bean soup, and chowders seem to take bran the best. You can add one and a half cups of water to each cup of condensed soup—instead of the usual one cup—when you use bran. The roughage thickens and extends the final product very nicely. If you think about it, bran costs hardly anything because it makes so many expensive foods go much farther.

Canned Dinners - These preparations are generally about as low in roughage as you can imagine, so added bran is very important. It is a welcome addition to dishes like spaghetti, noodles, lasagna, ravioli, beef stew, hash, chili con carne, goulash, pork and beans, meatballs and all the rest of the one-dish meals that come in cans.

Canned Vegetables - You have to use your own judgment here again. The vegetables that come in cream sauces, such as creamed corn, creamed onions, etc., take to bran easily. Most of the others do better if you make the kind of sauce described under "Frozen Foods" below.

Frozen Foods - The frozen foods that are most receptive to bran are the various frozen vegetables that come with more or less exotic sauces. You can add the usual, almost standard, one tablespoon of bran per person as soon as there is enough liquid melted in the cooking pot to absorb it. If you serve the kinds of frozen vegetables that don't have their own sauce, you can use this sauce over them:

One tablespoon bran
One tablespoon bread crumbs
Two tablespoons melted butter, margarine, or olive oil
Two tablespoons lemon juice

This is enough sauce for one person, and as usual, it supplies half the roughage requirement for that day.

Dry Mixes - If you like to use the various "helpers" for tuna, hamburger, and such dishes simply add about 1/4 cup of bran to each package. That provides half the daily roughage requirement for each person. Just be sure to use enough liquid to soften the bran—that usually means a bit more than the package instructions specify.

The other kinds of dry mixes—the ones you add for making goulash, stroganoff, stew, spaghetti sauce, chili con carne, sloppy Joes, Spanish rice, and similar dishes when you're really in a rush—can be enriched with about two ounces of bran to each package.

Seasoned Breadings - Those little packets of spices and things that you shake over chops and chicken before you bake them can be made much more healthful if you add up to 1/3 cup of bran to them and mix well before using. When you use your bran this way, you may want to put it in the blender at high speed for a few seconds to make the flakes smaller. You don't need to do it for any of the other types of recipes, but you'll find the breading adheres better if you take the extra time.

Pastry Mixes - Cake mixes, pancake and waffle mixes, instant stuffings, and similar products can be supplemented with bran very nicely. Just use the familiar one tablespoon per serving—and bear in mind that bran will be more obvious in some recipes than others. Angel food cake, for example, becomes much more nutritious and less harmful with bran, but it won't be the same angel food cake you have been used to. On the other hand, about 90 percent of the ready-mix flour products will be delightfully enhanced by the addition of bran.

Once you really get started restoring roughage to your family's diet, I think you'll become enthusiastic about it. You'll know that you're giving your loved ones the very best you possibly can and you'll see very quickly that it doesn't make cooking any more difficult. As a matter of fact, you can just measure out the entire bran ration for the whole family first thing in the morning and put it in a small bowl on the kitchen counter. As you go through the day, you can supplement various dishes with it until it's all used up. No matter how you do it, after a week or so, you'll find restoring the roughage to your family's daily diet will become second nature.

On those days when you find yourself with plenty of time on your hands—if that ever really happens any more—there are some wonderful recipes made with bran that are really worthwhile. Not only are they tasty and filling, but you'll have the satisfaction of eating the way people used to eat before all that essential roughage was taken away from them. There's just one little detail to remember: sometimes for one reason or another, a member of your family may not get enough of his or her daily roughage requirement this way. If that happens, simply supplement it with extra bran until he or she has the desired results as described in Chapter 7.

Here are some nice tasty recipes to start off with:

Eleven Main Dishes

Stuffed Pork Chops

6 pork chops, cut 1½ to 2 inches thick
Stuffing:
½ cup butter ¼ cup minced onions
1 tablespoon minced parsley
½ cup bread crumbs
¾ cup bran
¼ teaspoon black pepper
½ teaspoon sage
½ teaspoon thyme
2 tablespoons lemon juice
Salt to taste

DAILY REQUIREMENT FOR 6. SERVES 6

"Butterfly" each pork chop to make a pocket. Fill the chop with a stuffing made as follows:

Melt butter in a skillet. Sauté onions until transparent. Add parsley and bread crumbs and sauté a bit more. Remove from fire. Add the remaining ingredients. Mix well. Fill each pork-chop with 3 to 4 tablespoons of the mixture. Brown the chops in a skillet in 2 tablespoons of butter. Cover and let them cook slowly for 20 minutes. Serve with baked apple and brown rice.

Baked Stuffed Fish

Stuffing:
½ cup chopped onion
½ cup mushrooms, cut up
½ cup chopped celery
1 cup (2 sticks) butter
1 cup bran

2 cups bread crumbs

2 teaspoons parsley

½ teaspoon rosemary, tarragon, or marjoram

4 tablespoons lemon juice

Salt and pepper to taste

5-to-7-pound fish

DAILY REQUIREMENT FOR 8. SERVES 8.

Sauté onions, mushrooms, and celery in butter until onions become transparent. Put bran and bread crumbs in a mixing bowl. Add onion mixture, herbs, and lemon juice to bread-crumb mixture.

Wash the fish inside and out with cold water. Dry well, and rub the inside of the fish with a little salt. Spoon in the stuffing, packing lightly. Skewer or sew opening closed. Place fish in greased shallow ovenproof pan or place on greased aluminum foil in a shallow roasting pan. Brush the top of the fish with oil or lemon butter or cover with bacon strips or slices of salt pork. Bake at 350° for about 50 minutes or until the fish flakes easily with a fork. If you brush with a lemon butter mixture, baste with it occasionally. Suitable for red snapper, lake trout, bluefish, bass, shad, pike, carp, haddock, whitefish.

Variation - Use fish fillets and put the stuffing between two fillets or roll the fillets with stuffing. Brush with oil or lemon butter and bake same as above for 30 to 35 minutes or until the fish flakes easily with a fork.

Beef Stroganoff

1 tablespoon flour

2 tablespoons butter

2 cups beef stock

½ pint sour cream

2 tablespoons tomato juice or sauce

1 pound beef tenderloin, ½ inch thick cut into ½ x 2 inch strips

Salt and pepper to taste

1 cup bran

3 tablespoons butter

3 tablespoons minced onion

½ pound mushrooms, sliced
Pinch of nutmeg
DAILY REQUIREMENT FOR 8. SERVES 8

In a saucepan over gentle heat blend the flour with 2 tablespoons of butter until the mixture bubbles and is smooth. Stir in 2 cups of beef stock and cook until the mixture thickens. Add the sour cream and the tomato juice or sauce, stirring constantly. Add nutmeg and bran. Add a little milk to reduce the thickness of the sauce.

In the frying pan, melt 3 tablespoons of butter and fry the onion, mushrooms, and strips of beef sprinkled with black pepper. Cook about 5 minutes, turning so that the meat browns on all sides. Pour the meat mixture into the sauce and simmer gently for about 15 minutes. DO NOT BOIL. Serve with brown rice or flat egg noodles.

Easy Pizza Dough with Bran

Use a biscuit mix and follow the recipe on the label for pizza dough.

Add 1 cup of bran to the dough and a little more of the liquid to make the dough soft.

Make 2 pies. (If the pies are cut into eighths, 2 pieces equals the daily requirement of bran.)

Meat Sauce for Pizza with Bran

Mix 1 pound of ground meat with 1 egg and 1 cup of bran and a little tomato juice to moisten the meat. Spread on top of the pizza dough with cut-up tomatoes and grated cheese. Sprinkle top with Parmesan cheese. Bake at 400° for 25 to 30 minutes. (If the pies are cut into eighths, 2 pieces of meat sauce with bran contains the daily requirement.)

Macaroni and Cheese

2½ cups cooked macaroni, preferably whole-wheat macaroni
3 cups muenster or cheddar cheese
4 tablespoons minced onions

1 cup bran
2 cups thin white sauce (see recipe below)
DAILY REQUIREMENT FOR 8. SERVES 8.

Butter a 2-quart casserole. Put half of macaroni in casserole with half of the cheese and half of the onions and bran. Add remaining macaroni and top with the remaining cheese and onions and bran. Pour over the thin white sauce. Dot with butter. Bake at 3750 about 30 minutes or until lightly browned.

Thin White Sauce

2 tablespoons butter
1 tablespoon flour
2 cups milk

Melt butter. Blend in flour. Cook over low heat until smooth and bubbly. Remove from heat. Add milk. Return to the stove and heat to boiling, stirring constantly. Boil 1 minute. Remove from heat and add salt and pepper.

Beef Stew

2 large onions, chopped
¼ cup butter or oil
2 pounds cubed beef
6 to 8 cups beef broth
3 medium potatoes, pared and cubed
4 large carrots, peeled and quartered
1 cup fresh green beans
1 cup bran

Sauté onions in butter. Add meat and brown on all sides. Add enough broth to cover. Cover the pan and simmer 1½ to 2 hours. Add potatoes, carrots, beans, and bran. Add more liquid to cover if necessary. Simmer another half an hour.

Meat Loaf

1½ pounds ground beef (or 1 pound ground beef, ¼ pound ground veal, ¼ pound ground pork)
1 cup fine bread crumbs

¾ cup bran

1 egg

2 cloves garlic, minced, or 1 teaspoon powdered garlic
(or more to taste)

1 tablespoon Worcestershire sauce

1 tablespoon dry mustard

½ teaspoon sage

½ teaspoon thyme

Salt and pepper to taste

1 cup milk plus

DAILY REQUIREMENT FOR 6. SERVES 6.

Mix above ingredients together well, moistening with as much milk as necessary for a soft mixture. Put the mixture into a 9 x 5 x 3 ungreased loaf pan, dot with butter, and bake at 350° for 1¼ to 1½ hours.

Variation - Italian-Style Meat Loaf: Leave out milk, Worcestershire sauce, mustard, sage and thyme. Instead, add 1 tablespoon oregano, ½ teaspoon fennel seed, ¼ cup grated Parmesan cheese, a 1-pound can of whole canned tomatoes, and enough liquid to moisten well. Pour the rest of the liquid over top of loaf, sprinkle with Parmesan cheese, and dot with butter. Bake same as above.

Hamburgers

2 pounds ground meat

2 eggs

¼ cup minced onions

¾ cup bran

Salt and pepper to taste

DAILY REQUIREMENT FOR 6. SERVES 6.

Mix ingredients together well. Moisten with a little milk if necessary. Make into 6 hamburgers. Broil.

Variations:

Meatballs: Use above recipe, but make into small balls and fry in oil or butter.

Oriental hamburgers or meatballs: Add 2 tablespoons soy sauce, 1 teaspoon powdered ginger, 1 tablespoon sherry, 1 teaspoon powdered garlic.

Italian: Add ½ tablespoon oregano, ¼ teaspoon fennel seed, 2 tablespoons Parmesan cheese and moisten with a little tomato juice or sauce.

Quick Spaghetti Sauce

¼ cup olive oil
2 medium onions, finely chopped
1 pound of ground beef
1 can (1 pound, 12 ounces) whole tomatoes, undrained (sieved or blended)
1 can (8-ounce size) tomato sauce
1 cup bran
¼ cup Parmesan cheese
1 bay leaf
1 tablespoon dried basil leaves or 1 tablespoon oregano
½ teaspoon fennel seed
½ teaspoon black pepper
Fresh or powdered garlic to taste
¼ cup red wine or 2 tablespoons lemon juice
DAILY REQUIREMENT FOR 8. SERVES 8.

Sauté onions until slightly browned; add ground beef and brown. Add tomatoes, tomato sauce, bran, cheese, and spices. Add 1/4 cup Italian wine or 2 tablespoons of lemon juice. Simmer 15 minutes. Serve over spaghetti.

Stuffed Squash

1 large summer squash (12 to 14 inches long) or 2 medium-sized squash
1 pound ground beef
2 small onions, finely chopped
1 cup bran
6 to 8 whole canned tomatoes, drained (1- pound-12-ounce can)

1 egg
¼ cup Parmesan cheese Fresh or powdered garlic to taste
½ teaspoon black pepper ½ tablespoon dried oregano leaves
½ teaspoon crushed fennel seed
Juice from the 1-pound-12- ounce can of tomatoes
Butter

DAILY REQUIREMENT FOR 8. SERVES 8.

Cut the squash lengthwise and remove the seeds (Do not peel the squash.) In a bowl, mix well together the onions, bran, tomatoes, egg, cheese, and spices moistened with 8 to 10 tablespoons of the tomato juice from the canned tomatoes. Fill the squash and mound up the meat mixture. Place in a roasting pan with the remaining tomato juice and enough water to bring the liquid up to about an inch from the bottom. Sprinkle the tops with extra Parmesan cheese and dot in several places with butter. Bake at 375° for about 1 hour or until squash is tender.

Chili Con Carne

1 medium onion, chopped
2 tablespoons oil or bacon fat
1 pound ground beef
1 teaspoon powdered garlic or 4 cloves fresh garlic, crushed
2 cups cooked or canned kidney beans or chili beans
2 cups cooked or canned whole tomatoes
¾ cup bran
1 tablespoon chili powder or ground chili
½ teaspoon oregano
½ teaspoon cumin
Salt and pepper to taste

DAILY REQUIREMENT FOR 6. SERVES 6.

Fry onions in oil or bacon fat for about 1 minute. Add meat and garlic and fry, stirring constantly, about 3 minutes: Add beans, tomatoes, bran, and remaining spices. Cover and simmer 20 minutes.

Variation - Put bean-meat mixture into a 1-to-1½-quart casserole dish and top with corn-bread batter. Bake at 375° for 30 minutes.

Corn-Bread Batter

In a bowl mix:
1 cup stone-ground corn meal
½ teaspoon baking soda
1 tablespoon shortening, melted
1 egg
1 cup milk or buttermilk
Beat well and spoon over casserole.

Quick Breads

Drop Biscuits

2 cups flour (preferably stone-ground whole-wheat flour)
2 teaspoons baking powder
½ teaspoon salt
4 tablespoons butter
2 cups milk
1½ cups bran

Sift flour, baking powder, and salt together. Blend the butter into the flour mixture until the mixture looks like coarse meal. (You can blend with a pastry cutter or with 2 knives, cutting the butter into pea-sized pieces.) Add milk and bran alternately, stirring it in little by little. Drop by spoonful's onto a greased cookie sheet. Bake at 400° for 12 to 15 minutes.

Variation:

Cheese Biscuits: Add ½ cup grated cheese before adding milk.
3 DAYS' DAILY REQUIREMENT FOR 4 PEOPLE

Bran Muffins

1 cup flour (100% stone-ground whole-wheat flour)

1 teaspoon baking soda

1½ cups bran

½ cup raisins

1 egg, well-beaten

1 ½ cups molasses or honey

¾ cup milk

2 tablespoons soft butter or shortening

Put together dry ingredients and raisins and moisten with egg and molasses or honey, milk, and shortening. Stir only enough to blend. Bake in well-greased muffin tins at 400° for 20 to 30 minutes.

Dumplings

For beef or chicken stews or hearty vegetable and meat soups

1 cup flour (preferably 100% stone-ground whole-wheat flour)

2 teaspoons minced parsley

1 teaspoon grated onion

1¾ cup plus 2 teaspoons

½ cup bran milk

1/4 teaspoon salt

DAILY REQUIREMENT FOR 4. SERVES 4.

Mix all ingredients well. Drop from a teaspoon into stew. Cover and let simmer 15 minutes.

Breading

For fried chicken, veal cutlets, shrimp, pork chops, etc. Use half bran and half bread crumbs or half bran and half whole-wheat flour. If desired, bran may be processed quickly in blender, for this recipe only.

Banana Nut Bread

½ cup butter

¾ cup honey

2 eggs

2¼ cups flour (preferably whole-wheat pastry flour)

1 cup bran

2 teaspoons baking powder

½ cup milk with 1 tablespoon vinegar and ¼ teaspoon baking soda added

1 cup 2 to 3 large mashed bananas

½ teaspoon vanilla

1 cup chopped pecans (optional)

DAILY REQUIREMENT FOR 1 PERSON IS 4½ SLICES ¼ INCH THICK.

Cream butter and honey. Add eggs. Beat well after each addition. Mix flour, bran, and baking powder together. Add flour to butter mixture alternately with milk mixture. Add mashed bananas, vanilla, and nuts (if desired). Bake in a 9-by-5-by-3-inch loaf pan, well-greased and bottom lined with waxed paper, for 1 hour and 40 minutes at 325°.

Pancakes

Blend in a blender or beat the following:

1 cup whole-wheat pastry

3 eggs

2 cups milk

½ teaspoons vanilla

DAILY REQUIREMENT FOR 8

Blend at high speed or beat. Add more milk as needed to bring to heavy cream consistency. Butter skillet or griddle. Makes thin, light pancakes. Can be filled with sour cream or berries and topped with a bit of honey or sprinkled with raw natural sugar.

Waffles

In a blender put the following:

2 eggs

¼ cup salad oil or melted butter

2 cups milk

1½ cups whole-wheat pastry flour

1 cup bran

2 teaspoons baking powder

1 tablespoon honey

DAILY REQUIREMENT IS 2 WAFFLE SECTIONS PER PERSON.

Blend at high speed or beat well. Add more milk to thin, if necessary, to the consistency of heavy cream.

A rectangular waffle iron with four waffle sections makes 16 individual waffle sections.

High-Fiber Crackers

1 cup bran

1¼ cups gluten flour

1½ cups milk

½ cup sesame seeds

1 cup water

¼ cup stone-ground whole-Wheat flour

½ teaspoon baking soda

1 teaspoon salt

5 CRACKERS ARE DAILY REQUIREMENT FOR 1, 3 GRAMS ROUGHAGE PER CRACKER.

Put all the ingredients into a mixing bowl and mix well. A soft dough will form. Lightly flour a board or counter top and roll the dough out until it is 1/8 inch thick. Score the dough with a knife into 2 x 4" rectangles. Place on a well greased baking sheet. Bake in a preheated oven at 350° for 10 minutes. Then lower the temperature to 300° and leave another 10 minutes or so until the dough is crisp like a cracker. Makes forty crackers.

For onion flavor–add 2 tablespoons of dried minced onion to above.

For garlic flavor–add 2 tablespoons of powdered garlic.

For cheese flavor–add 2 tablespoons of grated Parmesan or Romano cheese.

Bread Stuffing

2 medium onions, finely chopped

2 cups celery chopped, stalks and leaves

1 cup butter

8 cups small bread cubes (preferably whole wheat bread)
1 1/2 cups bran
2 1/2 teaspoons sage
1/2 teaspoons thyme
1 teaspoon pepper
Salt to taste

DAILY REQUIREMENT FOR TWELVE PEOPLE

Fry onions and celery in 1 cup butter until tender. In a large bowl combine the onions and celery mixture, the small bread cubes, the bran, and the spices. Makes enough for a 10 to 12 pound turkey.

Use the above stuffing recipe with the following changes for a variety of stuffing all containing bran.

Cornbread stuffing - bread cubes should be half cornbread, half regular bread.

Mushroom stuffing - add 1/2 cup mushrooms sautéed with onions to every cup of bread cubes. Reduce bread cubes to 6 cups. For recipe above, 3 cups of mushrooms are needed.

Sausage stuffing - add 1 pound of sausage meat crumbled and browned.

Giblet stuffing - simmer the heart, the gizzard, and the neck from the chicken or turkey in broth with a dash of pepper, thyme, sage, and salt to taste for about an hour. Add the liver during the last 10 minutes. Chop these ingredients (except the neck) and add to the above ingredients.

Pecan stuffing - reduce the bread cubes to 6 cups and add 2 cups of chopped pecans.

Chestnut stuffing - reduce the bread cubes to 6 cups. Leave out the celery. Reduce the amount of onion to one small onion, sautéed in 1/2 cup butter with 1 tablespoon of chopped parsley. Leave out the sage and thyme. Add pepper and salt to taste and 1 cup cooked or canned chestnuts.

Yeast Bread Dough

(for rolls or loaves)

1 ½ cups milk
1½ teaspoons honey

¼ pound (1 stick) butter or ½ cup shortening

½ cup honey

2 eggs

2 packages active dry yeast*

4 to 6 cups of stone-ground whole-wheat flour

2 cups gluten flour

2 cups bran

* Into ¼ cup warm water (105 to 115°F); put 2 packages of yeast with a dash of sugar. Let stand five to ten minutes.

DAILY REQUIREMENT FOR 1 PERSON IS 4½ SLICES OF BREAD ¼ INCH THICK.

Scald milk. Add butter and honey and let cool. In a mixing bowl put 2 eggs and the cooled milk mixture. Add 2 cups of whole-wheat flour and start to beat. Add the yeast dissolved in water and 2 cups of gluten flour. Beat. Add 2 cups bran and beat again. When the dough becomes too stiff to beat with regular beaters (if your machine has a dough hook, you can do the entire operation in the mixing bowl), turn it out onto a floured bread-board or countertop and start to knead. Knead in as much of the rest of the whole-wheat flour as you need to have moderately soft, unsticky dough. To hand-knead the bread takes about 20 minutes. (With the dough hook, it only takes about 5 to 7 minutes.) Place kneaded dough in a large, well-oiled deep bowl or pan covered with a towel and left in a warm place. Let rise until double in bulk—about 1½ to 2 hours. Punch down. Make into 2 loaves and place in well-oiled loaf pans. Cover and let rise again in a warm place for about an hour—until almost doubled. Dough will rise up over the pan. Place in a preheated oven set at 350° for 40 minutes. Turn loaves out of pan and let cool on their sides. Each loaf contains 1 cup of bran.

If rolls are desired, place balls of dough about 1 inch apart in well-greased pie plates or shallow cake pans— or put 3 small balls in each well-greased muffin tin. Let rise about an hour. Bake in preheated 425° oven for 10 minutes.

Five Delicious Desserts

Hi-Roughage Rice Pudding

¼ cup uncooked brown rice

4 cups milk

1 tablespoon cinnamon

½ cup honey

¾ cup bran

1 teaspoon vanilla

½ cup raisins

DAILY REQUIREMENT FOR 6. SERVES 6.

In an 8-by-8-inch baking pan or Pyrex pan mix all of the above ingredients. Bake at 275° to 300° for 3 hours. Stir a few times during the first hour.

Variation - Use cracked wheat or buckwheat groats (kasha) instead of rice.

Apple Brown Betty

2 cups bread crumbs

¾ cup bran

1/3 cup melted butter

6 cups cored, peeled, and sliced apples (7 to 8 medium)

½ cup honey

1 teaspoon cinnamon or ¼ teaspoon nutmeg

Grated rind of ½ lemon

Juice of 1 lemon

¼ cup water.

Mix together bread crumbs, bran, and butter. In another bowl, mix well: apples, honey, cinnamon, grated lemon rind, and half of the lemon juice. In a 6-to-8-cup buttered casserole dish put a layer of ½ of the bread-crumb mixture, then a layer of half the apple mixture, another layer of the bread-crumb mixture, the remaining apple mixture, and top with remaining bread-crumb mixture. Pour the remaining lemon juice mixed with water over the top. Dot with butter. Bake covered in a preheated oven at 350° for 20 minutes.

Then uncover for remaining 15 minutes. Serve hot or cold with whipped cream.

Chocolate Chip Cookies

1 cup butter
1 cup honey
1 teaspoon vanilla
2 eggs
2¼ cups whole-wheat pastry flour
1 cup bran
1 teaspoon baking soda
¼ cup water
12-ounce package chocolate bits

9½ COOKIES CONTAIN THE DAILY REQUIREMENT

Cream butter; add the honey and beat. Add the vanilla and eggs and beat well. Mix the flour, bran, and baking soda together and add this mixture alternately with water. Beat well after each addition. Add the chocolate bits. Mix the bits into batter well. Drop by spoonfuls onto a greased baking sheet. Bake at 375° for 7 to 8 minutes. Makes 75 1½-inch cookies.

Date-Nut Torte

3 eggs, separated
16 dates, pitted and chopped
2 tablespoons whole-wheat pastry flour
½cup bran
½ cup chopped pecans
1 teaspoon baking powder
¼ cup honey

DAILY REQUIREMENT FOR 4. SERVES 4.

Beat the egg yolks. Add the dates, nuts, honey, flour, bran, and baking powder. In a separate bowl beat egg whites until stiff. Fold the egg whites into the date mixture. Pour into a greased 8-inch pie plate and bake at 350° for 20 minutes.

Brownies

¾ cup flour (whole-wheat pastry flour)

½ teaspoon baking powder

1 teaspoon vanilla

½ cup butter

3 eggs

¾ cup honey

½ cup bran

2 squares unsweetened baking chocolate

4 SQUARES EQUAL THE DAILY REQUIREMENT FOR I PERSON.

Measure flour and mix in baking powder. In a small pan or double boiler, melt ½ cup butter with chocolate. Put eggs into a mixing bowl and beat until light and fluffy. Add honey and beat well again. Add chocolate-butter mixture, beating continuously. Add vanilla. Add flour mixture and bran slowly, beating slowly. Beat only enough to blend. Pour into greased 8-inch square pan. Bake at 350° for 15 to 20 minutes. Do not overbake. Cut into 2-inch-square pieces, this recipe mikes a total of 16 pieces.

Variation - Add ¾ cup chopped walnuts or pecans.

As you continue to use bran and high-roughage cereals in your daily menu planning, I'm sure you will develop some of your own exciting and delicious ways to restore roughage to your family's diet.

I hope you enjoyed this book and my fervent wish is that it brings you and your family health and happiness every day of your lives.

Made in United States
Orlando, FL
11 February 2023